Critical Care

&

Emergency Guide

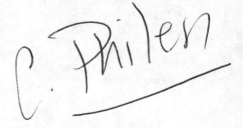

C. Philen

Critical Care

&

Emergency Guide

Craig A. Kizewic, DO
St. Vincent Mercy Medical Center
Emergency Medicine
Ohio University College of
Osteopathic Medicine

Critical Care Transport Nurse
St. Vincent & Medical College
LifeFlight / Mobile Life
Critical Care Transport Network

First Edition

ISBN
1-929925-80-8

Craig A. Kizewic, DO
Critical Care & Emergency Guide

FIRSTPUBLISH, INC.
300 Sunport Ln.
Orlando, FL 32809
407-240-1414
www.firstpublish.com

Printed By QUESTprint
Orlando, Florida

NOTICE

Medicine is an ever-changing science and as such, we must all attempt to broaden our knowledge as new research and clinical experience guides us throughout our lives. This pocketbook is intended to be used as a quick overview, reference and reminder of what you have already learned through your years of education. It is certainly not all-inclusive. The accuracy and completeness of this work cannot be guaranteed. I have attempted to incorporate the most recent data and medication recommendations. Exhaustive efforts were put forth to make this book as accurate as possible. However, being only human, errors can and will occur. Therefore, no one affiliated with this work warrants that the information contained herein is in every respect accurate or complete, nor is anyone affiliated with this work responsible for any errors or omissions or for the results obtained from use of the information in this book. This book is not intended to be a replacement for experience, medical education and training, or continuing medical education.

ACKNOWLEDGEMENTS

I would like to thank my parents and family for all of the love, support and patience throughout the years of my medical education through both nursing and medical school. Without their unconditional love, understanding and rearing, I would certainly not be the person who I am today. I would further like to thank the reviewers of this book, Kathy Justus, RN, CNNP, who instructed me in Neonatal Resuscitation and was my mentor during my rotation in Pediatrics; to my best friend Kimberly A. Beauch, BIS-NS, RN, EMT-A, who has always been there for me. You are a true friend and dearly loved. To Stewart Isley, the other three musketeer, who is now in medical school and loving every minute of it. He is eagerly waiting to start his fourth year rotations and will be pursuing a career in Emergency Medicine.

Simple words are not enough for how I cherish these people who have loved, supported and guided me throughout the years. They all hold a special place in my heart and I am eternally grateful to each of them for the special things that they have taught me in life and for the things I will continue to learn as my life progresses.

I would also like to thank the many instructors throughout the years of my nursing education, medical school education, and residency for sharing their knowledge and experiences which help those pursuing careers in a medical field, to become a better nurse or physician. Your time, sharing of knowledge and commitment to the profession are greatly appreciated.

V

ACTION POTENTIAL

Phase 0: Rapid Upstroke – Na$^+$ enters cell causing (+) charge. Results in depolarization. Seen as P-wave or QRS complex.

Phase 1: Partial Repolarization – Cell becomes slightly less (+). Na$^+$ channels close, K$^+$ channels begin to open.

Phase 2: Plateau – Cell isoelectric. Slow Ca^{++} channels open resulting in the influx of Ca^{++} which is balanced by K$^+$ efflux. Seen as ST- segment.

Phase 3: Rapid Repolarization – K$^+$ moves out of cell via slow K$^+$ channels. Closure of Ca^{++} channels. Results in repolarization. Seen as T-wave.

Phase 4: Resting Potential – Na$^+$ pumped out of the cell and K$^+$ moves into cell as a result of the Na$^+$/K$^+$ pump. Energy needed for pump comes from ATP.

- -

ADVANCED CARDIAC LIFE SUPPORT

VF/Pulseless VT

- ABC's
- CPR
- Defibrillate 200 J, 300 J, 360 J
- CPR
- Intubate
- Obtain IV access
- Epinephrine 1 mg IV q 3 – 5 min
                    OR
- Vasopressin 40 U IV
  *Single dose ONLY
- Defibrillate 360 J after each medication
- Consider antiarrhythmics
  - Amiodarone (IIb): 300 mg IV
    *If arrest recurs, consider administering a second dose of 150 mg IV
    *MAX: 2.2 g over 24 hrs
  - Lidocaine (Indeterminate): 1.0 – 1.5 mg/kg IV
    *MR in 3 – 5 min to MAX of 3 mg/kg
  - $MgSO_4$ 1 – 2 g IV
    *Use for polymorphic VT (Torsades de Pointes or suspected hypomagnesemia (IIb)
  - Procainamide 17 mg/kg @ 30 mg/min
    *Use for intermittent or recurrent VF/Pulseless VT (IIb)

- Consider NaHCO$_3$ 1 mEq/kg IV
  Class I:
    - Known, preexisting
      hyperkalemia
  Class IIa:
    - Preexisting bicarbonate-
      responsive acidosis
    - OD w/ TCA
    - Alkalinize the urine in drug OD
  Class IIb:
    - Intubated and continued long
      arrest
    - Upon return of spontaneous
      circulation after prolonged
      arrest
  Class III:
    - Hypoxic lactic acidosis

- Resume defibrillation at 360 J if rhythm
  has not converted

*Class I: definitely helpful
Class IIa: acceptable, probably helpful
Class IIb: acceptable, possibly helpful
Class III: not indicated, may be harmful

(con't)

ACLS (con't)
Pulseless Electrical Activity (PEA)
- ABC's
- CPR
- Differential diagnosis and treat
  appropriately:
  - Hypovolemia (#1 cause)
  - Hypoxia
  - Hypothermia
  - Hydrogen ion – acidosis
  - Hyper-/hypokalemia
  - Thrombosis, pulmonary
    (embolism)
  - Tension pneumothorax
  - Thrombosis, coronary (ACS)
  - Tamponade, cardiac
  - "Tablets" (drug OD)
- Epinephrine 1 mg IV q 3 – 5 min
- Atropine 1 mg IV q 3 – 5 min if absolute
  or relative bradycardia
  *MAX: 0.04 mg/kg

Asystole
- ABC's
- CPR
- Confirm true asystole in > 1 lead
- Differential diagnosis and treat
  appropriately:
  - Hypoxia
  - Hypothermia
  - Hyper-/hypokalemia
  - Hydrogen ion - acidosis

- Thrombosis, coronary (ACS)
- "Tablets" (drug OD)
- TCP
  *If considered, perform immediately
- Epinephrine 1 mg IV q 3 – 5 min
- Atropine 1 mg IV q 3 – 5 min
  MAX: 0.04 mg/kg
- Consider termination of efforts
  *Consider quality of resuscitation?
  *Atypical clinical features present?
  *Support for cease-efforts protocols in place?

*"Asystole most often represents a confirmation of death rather than a 'rhythm' to be treated." (From *Circulation*, American Heart Association, 2000, p. 1-154)

Bradycardia
- ABC's, IV, VS, 12-lead, PCXR, etc.
- Serious S/S
  - Atropine 0.5 – 1.0 mg IV q 3 – 5 min to MAX of 0.03 – 0.04 mg/kg
  - TCP if available
    *If the patient is symptomatic, DO NOT delay TCP while awaiting IV access or for atropine to take effect
  - Dopamine: 5 – 20 µg/kg/min
  - Epinephrine: 2 – 10 µg/min

(con't)

ACLS – Bradycardia (con't)

*If 2° AVB or 3° AVB, prepare for TCP.
Should symptoms develop, use TCP as a
bridge until TVP is inserted.

*Cardiac transplant patients ∅ respond to
atropine, therefore go immediately to TCP
and/or catecholamine infusion

Tachycardias
- ABC's, IV, VS, 12-lead, PCXR, etc.

*If patient becomes symptomatic throughout
any of the treatment, immediately use
synchronized cardioversion and premedicate
whenever possible:
- PSVT: start @ 100 J
- Atrial flutter: start @ 100 J
- Atrial fibrillation: start @ 100 J
- Ventricular tachycardia: start @ 100 J

- **Atrial Fibrillation or Flutter**
    - **Rate Control**
        - <u>Heart Function Preserved</u>
            - Use **one** of the following:
                - Diltiazem
                - β-blockers
                - Verapamil
                - Amiodarone

- <u>Impaired Heart</u>
  *EF < 40% or CHF
  - Use **one** of the following:
    - Digoxin (IIb)
    - Diltiazem (IIb)
    - Amiodarone (IIb)

- **Convert Rhythm**
  - <u>Heart Function Preserved</u>
  - *Duration < 48 hrs*
    - Consider DC cardioversion
    - Use **one** of the following:
      - Amiodarone (IIa)
      - Ibutilide (IIa)
      - Flecainide (IIa)
      - Propafenone (IIa)
      - Procainamide (IIa)
      - Sotalol (IIb)
      - Disopyramide (IIb)

  - <u>Impaired Heart</u>
    *EF < 40% or CHF
  - *Duration < 48 hrs*
    - Consider DC cardioversion
      OR
    - Amiodarone (IIb)

(con't)

ACLS – Tachy – Af/AF (con't)

- <u>Heart Function Preserved</u>
- *Duration > 48 hrs*
    - Delayed Cardioversion
        - NO DC cardioversion
        - Anticoagulate for 3 weeks
        - Cardiovert
        - Anticoagulate an additional 4 weeks
        OR
    - Early Cardioversion
        - Begin IV heparin immediately
        - TEE to exclude atrial clot
        - Cardiovert within 24 hrs
        - Anticoagulate for additional 4 weeks

- <u>Impaired Heart</u>
  *EF < 40% or CHF
- *Duration > 48 hrs*
    - Anticoagulation as above
    - DC cardioversion

- **Atrial Fibrillation or Flutter with WPW**
  - **Rate Control**
    - <u>Heart Function Preserved</u>
      - DC cardioversion
        OR
      - Use **one** of the following:
        - Amiodarone (IIb)
        - Flecainide (IIb)
        - Procainamide (IIb)
        - Propafenone (IIb)
        - Sotalol (IIb)

      *III (Can Be Harmful)
      - Adenosine
      - β-blockers
      - Ca^{++} channel blockers
      - Digoxin

    - <u>Impaired Heart</u>
      *EF < 40% or CHF
      - DC cardioversion
        OR
      - Amiodarone (IIb)

(con't)

ACLS – Tachy – Af/AF w/ WPW (con't)
- **Convert Rhythm**
  - *Duration < 48 hrs*
    - DC cardioversion
      OR
    - Use **one** of the following:
      - Amiodarone (IIb)
      - Flecainide (IIb)
      - Procainamide (IIb)
      - Propafenone (IIb)
      - Sotalol (IIb)

      *III (Can Be Harmful)
      - Adenosine
      - β-blockers
      - Ca^{++} channel blockers
      - Digoxin

  - *Duration > 48 hrs*
    - Anticoagulation as above
    - DC cardioversion

- **Narrow-Complex Supraventricular Tachycardia, Stable**
  - 12-Lead ECG to establish diagnosis
  - Attempt therapeutic diagnostic maneuver
    - Vagal stimulation
    - Adenosine

- **Junctional Tachycardia**
    - <u>Preserved</u>
        - **NO** DC cardioversion
        - Amiodarone
        - β-blocker
        - Ca^{++} channel blocker

    - <u>EF < 40% or CHF</u>
        - **NO** DC cardioversion
        - Amiodarone

- **PSVT**
    - <u>Preserved</u>
        - *Priority Order*:
            - Ca^{++} channel blockers
            - β-blockers
            - Digoxin
            - DC cardioversion
            - Consider
                - Procainamide
                - Amiodarone
                - Sotalol

    - <u>EF < 40% or CHF</u>
        - *Priority Order:*
            - **NO** DC cardioversion
            - Digoxin
            - Amiodarone
            - Diltiazem

(con't)

ACLS – Tachy – Narrow-Complex (con't)
- **Ectopic or MAT**
    - <u>Preserved</u>
        - **NO** DC cardioversion
        - Ca^{++} channel blockers
        - β-blockers
        - Amiodarone

    - <u>EF < 40% or CHF</u>
        - **NO** DC cardioversion
        - Amiodarone
        - Diltiazem

- **Wide-Complex Tachycardia: Unknown Type, Stable**
    - 12-Lead ECG to establish diagnosis
    - <u>Preserved</u>
        - DC cardioversion
            OR
        - Procainamide
            OR
        - Amiodarone

    - <u>EF < 40% or CHF</u>
        - DC cardioversion
            OR
        - Amiodarone

- **Ventricular Tachycardia, Stable**
  - **Monomorphic VT**
    - <u>Preserved</u>
      - Any **one** of the following:
        - Procainamide (IIa)
        - Sotalol (IIa)
        - Amiodarone (IIb)
        - Lidocaine (IIb)

    - <u>EF < 40% or CHF</u>
      - Amiodarone 150 mg IV bolus over 10 min q 10 – 15 min prn
        *Then use infusion
        *MAX in 24 hrs: 2.2 g
        OR
      - Lidocaine 0.5 – 0.75 mg/kg IV q 5 – 10 min to max of 3 mg/kg
        *Infuse 1 – 4 mg/min after bolus complete
      - Synchronized cardiovert

(con't)

- **Polymorphic VT**
  - <u>Normal QT Interval</u>
    - Treat ischemia
    - Correct electrolytes
    - Use **one** of the following:
      - β-blockers
      - Lidocaine
      - Amiodarone
      - Procainamide
      - Sotalol
    - Synchronized cardioversion

  - <u>Long QT Interval</u>
    - Correct abnormal electrolytes
    - Use **one** of the following:
      - Magnesium
      - Overdrive pacing
      - Isoproterenol
      - Phenytoin
      - Lidocaine

- - - - - - - - - - - - - - - - - - - -

AORTIC DISSECTION

S/S: Chest pain, aortic insufficiency, myocardial ischemia/infarction, uneven upper or lower extremity pulses, pericardial tamponade

Goal:
- Lower the blood pressure to a SBP < 120 mmHg w/o producing a paradoxic ↑ in HR or CO
- Blunt the shearing force of the blood against the aortic wall by ↓ cardiac contractility to a heart rate of approximately 60 beats per minute
- Control pain

*Common sites include the R lateral wall of the ascending aorta (site of high hydraulic shear stress) and the descending thoracic aorta just distal to the ligamentum arteriosum

Tx: Multi-drug therapy
- Propranolol 0.5 mg IV, then 1 mg IV q 15 min

OR

- Esmolol 500 µg/kg IV bolus followed by infusion

AND

- Nitroprusside 0.2 – 10 µg/kg/min

15 (con't)

Aortic Dissection (con't)

Tx: Monotherapy
- Labetalol 20 mg IV, then 1 – 2 mg/min
  OR
- Labetalol 20 mg IV, then 40 mg IV q 10 min

*Must give propranolol first to avoid a paradoxic ↑ in HR which leads to an ↑ in CO
Note: metoprolol may also be used

Stanford Classification:
- Type A: involves the ascending aorta – **surgical emergency**
- Type B: involves the transverse or descending aorta w/o involvement of the ascending aorta

- -

AV BLOCKS – SITE OF BLOCK

1° AVB – anywhere from AV node to bundle branches

2° AVB Type I – AV node

2° AVB Type II – Bundle of HIS or below

3° AVB – anywhere from AV node to bundle branches

- -

CARDIAC MURMURS – GRADING

I	Faintly audible; only heard w/ special effort
II	Faint; easily audible
III	Moderately loud
IV	Loud; associated w/ a thrill
V	Very loud; associated w/ a thrill; may be heard w/ stethoscope off the chest
VI	Maximum loudness; associated w/ a thrill; heard w/o a stethoscope

- -

ECG – 12-LEAD
AXIS DEVIATION (Quadrant Method):
1. Determine whether the QRS complex is mainly (+) or (−) in the following leads: I and aVF or I and II.
- If Lead I is (+) and lead aVF or Lead II is (+), then the patient has a normal axis deviation
- If Lead I is (+) and lead aVF or Lead II is (−), then the patient has a left axis deviation
- If Lead I is (−) and lead aVF or Lead II is (+), then the patient has a right axis deviation
- If Lead I is (−) and lead aVF or Lead II is (−), then the patient has an extreme right axis deviation

(con't)

17

ECG – 12-Lead – Axis Deviation (con't)
-   Use the following chart:

	Lead I	aVF or Lead II
Normal Axis	+	+
Left Axis	+	−
Right Axis	−	+
Extreme R Axis	−	−

Degrees of Axis Deviation

Normal Axis:	0 to + 90
Left Axis: Mild:	0 to − 30
Moderate:	− 30 to − 90
Right Axis:	+ 90 to + 180
Extreme R Axis:	− 90 to − 180

2.   Now that you have the quadrant, the degrees need to be narrowed further. To do this, find the most equiphasic lead. The axis will lie at a right angle to this lead.
-   If the equiphasic lead is Lead I, look at aVF. If aVF look at I.
-   If the equiphasic lead is Lead II, look at aVL. If aVL look at II.
-   If the equiphasic lead is Lead III, look at aVR. If aVR look at III.

3. To narrow the axis further, if the lead is not completely equiphasic, then move the axis proportionally to the (+) or (−) pole of the equiphasic lead. i.e. If the most equiphasic lead is slightly positive, move the axis toward the (+) pole of the lead you chose w/o entering the area of another lead. Do the opposite if the equiphasic lead is slightly more (−). This will be your axis.

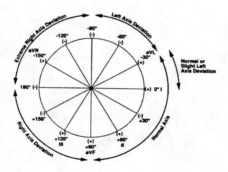

(From Brose, J., Waksman, D., Jarosick, M.: *The Pocket Guide to EKG Interpretation*, Ohio University, 1993.)

(con't)

ECG – 12-Lead (con't)
Causes of Axis Deviation
- Normal Axis: wnl

- Left Axis:
  - Mild: wnl, AMI, apical-ventricular aneurysm, LVH

  - Moderate: extensive IWMI, emphysema, WPW, RV pacemaker, hyperkalemia, LBBB, L anterior hemiblock, ventricular ectopy

- Right Axis: RVH, COPD, pulmonary HTN, L posterior hemiblock, extensive LWMI, WPW, RBBB, hyperkalemia, ventricular ectopy

- Extreme R Axis: VT

BUNDLE BRANCH BLOCKS
V1, V2 look at right side of heart
V5, V6 look at left side of heart

- T-wave should be in the opposite
  direction. If not, suspect myocardial
  ischemia.

- Incomplete blocks have a QRS
  morphology similar to RBBB or LBBB
  but the QRS is < 0.11

RBBB: V1: QRS > 0.11 w/ rSr' morphology
V6: QRS > 0.11

   Causes: AWMI, CAD, congenital
   anomalies, HTN

LBBB: V1: QRS > 0.12 w/ mainly (−) qS or
(−) rS
V6: QRS > 0.12 w/ rabbit ears

   Causes: IWMI, AWMI, coronary
   insufficiency, calcified aortic
   valve, HTN, RV pacemaker

(con't)

ECG – 12-Lead (con't)
HEMIBLOCKS
Can only be determined if there is no other reason for the axis deviation.

Left Anterior Fascicular Block
- LAD > − 40°
- Normal QRS duration
- Small r in II, III, aVF w/ deep S
- Small Q-wave in aVL

Causes: AMI (AWMI greater), HTN, aortic valve dz, cardiomyopathy

Left Posterior Fascicular Block
- RAD > +105°
- R in I, aVL (rS complex)
- qR complex in II, III, aVF

Causes: AMI, usually associated w/ RBBB

Bifascicular Block = RBBB + hemiblock
Trifasicular Block = 3° AVB

HYPERTROPHIES
LAH (P-Mitrale)
-    II: P-wave > 0.12, notched L > R, PLUS

-    V1: biphasic P-wave w/ R atrial
           depolarization slightly (+) and L
           atrial depolarization (–)

*Left atrium upper limit of wnl is 4.0 cm

Causes: Mitral stenosis, mitral insufficiency,
             poor LV function, aortic stenosis,
             aortic insufficiency

RAH (P-Pulmonale)
-    II: notched P-wave R > L or > 3 mm
           peaked or pointed P-wave which is
           often taller in III than in I

-    V1: biphasic P-wave R atrial
           depolarization (+) and L atrial
           depolarization slightly (–)

*Right atrium upper limit of wnl if 4.0 cm

Causes: Tricuspid valve stenosis, atrial-septal
             defect, pulmonary HTN, COPD,
             pulmonary embolus, left sided heart
             failure, myopathy

(con't)

23

ECG – 12-Lead – Hypertrophies (con't)
LVH
- R-wave in aVL + S-wave in V3 > 24 mm in males and > 20 mm in females

Causes: Aortic valve stenosis or insufficiency, HTN, CAD, chronic myocarditis, mitral insufficiency, myopathy

Look for LV strain = ST depression and T-wave inversion in lateral leads
*Normally the LV wall measures < 1.5 cm. If LV wall > 1.5 cm it indicates hypertrophy.

RVH
- progressive lessening of R-wave in V1 – V4   OR
- no change in R-wave in V1 – V4   OR
- R-wave > S-wave in V1   OR
- Large S-wave in V5 and V6

Causes: Pulmonary HTN, pulmonary valve stenosis or insufficiency, left sided heart failure, pulmonary embolus, COPD, myopathy

*ECG primarily detects LVH so RVH is **severe** when seen*
*Normally RV wall measures 0.3 – 0.5 cm. If RV wall > 0.5 cm it indicates hypertrophy.

PULMONARY EMBOLUS ECG CHANGES

- Sinus tachycardia – most common finding
- Tall P-wave in inferior leads (R atrial overload)
- S_I, Q_{III}, $\perp_{III}$: S-wave in Lead I, Q-wave in Lead III, T-wave inversion in Lead III
- S_I, S_{II}, S_{III}: S-wave in Lead I, S-wave in Lead II, S-wave in Lead III

- -

MYOCARDIAL INFARCTION

Sensitivity for detecting myocardial ischemia:

- Monitoring in V5 alone – 75%
- Monitoring in Lead II alone – 24%
- Monitoring in V5 and Lead II – 85%

- Maximum QT prolongation occurs 2 days post MI, therefore the patient is prone to arrhythmias including Torsades de Pointes

- The infarcted tissue is maximally soft by day 10 (4 – 10 days post MI), therefore patient is prone to ventricular free wall rupture, interventricular septal rupture, papillary muscle rupture and cardiac tamponade

(con't)

Myocardial Infarction (con't)
General Management of LVMI
1. Establish 2 IV's
2. Limit fluids
3. Initial medications
   - Oxygen
   - Nitroglycerin for pain and blood pressure control
   - ASA
   - Thrombolytic therapy
   - Heparin
   - Morphine for pain control
   - IV β-blockers unless HR < 60, CHF, SBP < 100, severe COPD, Type I and II 2° AVB and 3° AVB
   - ACE Inhibitor if large AWMI, LV dysfunction, EF < 40%, normotension
   - Consider magnesium
   - Consider stat cardiac catheterization if available or if the patient is not reperfusing
4. Continuous monitoring and reassessing

General Management of RVMI
1. Establish 2 IV's
2. Judicious use of fluids if needed for blood pressure control
3. Initial medications
   - Oxygen
   - ASA
   - Limit nitroglycerin, morphine and diuretics

- Heparin
- Thrombolytic therapy
- Dobutamine for hypotension unresponsive to fluids
- Consider stat cardiac catheterization if available or if the patient is not reperfusing

4. Continuous monitoring and reassessing

ANTERIOR WALL MI: Occlusion of LCA
*LCA supplies RBB, LBB, anterior 2/3 of ventricular septum

ECG: V1 – V2 (septal), V2 – V4 (anterior), V1 – V6 (extensive anterior)

Complications: CHF, cardiogenic shock, sinus tachycardia, VPB's, atrial arrhythmias, IVCD: RBBB or LBBB, 2° AVB Type II leading to 3° AVB

S/S: Ventricular gallop (S3), atrial gallop (S4), ↑ PCWP, pulmonary edema, CHF, shock
*3° AVB = 70 – 80% mortality if develops w/ an AMI

*Loss of R-wave progression in V1 – V6 indicates an extensive anterior or anterolateral infarction   (con't)

Myocardial Infarction (con't)
INFERIOR WALL MI: Occlusion of the RCA
*RCA supplies blood to the SA node in 55% of hearts and the AV node and Bundle of HIS in 90% of hearts
*RCA supplies the inferior portion of the LV via posterior descending artery in 80% of hearts which indicates R dominance
*AV blocks are common and are generally ischemic, transient and reversible

ECG: II, III, aVF

Complications: Sinus bradycardia, sinus arrest, exit blocks, N/V leading to vagal stimulation and syncope, bronchospasm, tracheal burning

S/S: N/V, bradycardia

*33 – 50% of IWMI's also have some RV involvement, therefore, obtain a right sided ECG to rule out RV infarction
*If RV infarct is present, the right sided ECG should show V_4R ST-segment elevation

Bezold-Jarish Reflex: Associated w/ an IWMI. NOT due to RV involvement. Patient becomes bradycardic w/ hypotension due to activation of mechanoreceptors. May be adenosine driven. Treatment is fluids and limiting nitrates.

LATERAL WALL MI: Occlusion of the marginal branch of the circumflex or diagonal branches of the LAD

*Circumflex supplies the SA node in 45% of hearts and the AV node in 10% of hearts

ECG: I, aVL, V5 – V6

Complications: Lateral wall involvement is frequently seen w/ extensive AWMI and occasionally w/ IWMI

S/S: MI in this site alone is uncommon. Look for PWMI w/ bradycardia and conduction defects.

POSTERIOR WALL MI: Occlusion of the RCA or, less commonly, a branch of the circumflex artery

ECG: Reciprocal changes in V1 – V3
- **ST-segment depression**
- **Tall symmetric T-waves**
- **Initial R-wave upswing is tall and broad**

(con't)

Myocardial Infarction – PWMI (con't)
Complications: Bradycardia, heart block
(usually transient)

RIGHT VENTRICULAR WALL MI: Occlusion
of the proximal segment of RCA in
combination w/ LV inferior infarct

ECG: V4R – V6R

*Morphology of V_4R w/ RVMI:
- **If elevated ST-segment =
proximal RCA occlusion**
- **If ST-segment coves into a
(+) T-wave = distal RCA
occlusion**
- **If ST-segment slopes into a
(–) T-wave = circumflex
occlusion**

Complications: Right sided heart failure
*Tx w/ volume loading and dobutamine

S/S: JVD, HJR, ↓ CO, hypotension, oliguria,
minimal to absent pulmonary congestion,
shock w/ peripheral vasoconstriction

*Use caution w/ morphine, NTG, diuretics
*33 – 50% of IWMI's also have some RV
involvement, therefore obtain a right sided
ECG to rule out RV infarction

- - - - - - - - - - - - - - - - - - - -

PACEMAKER BASIC NOMENCLATURE

Paced	Sensed	Mode	Activity
A	A	I	R
V	V	T	
D	D	D	

A = Atrium, V = Ventricle, D = Dual, R = Rate
response, I = Inhibited, T = Triggered

VVI = Ventricular demand pacemaker
AAI = Atrial chamber pacemaker
DDD = Dual chamber demand pacemaker

I = If pacemaker sees an event, it WILL NOT
put out a spike. e.g. VVI: if pacemaker
senses a ventricular depolarization, it will
NOT put out the ventricular spike.

T = If pacemaker sees an event, it WILL put
out a spike. e.g. DDD: if pacemaker
senses an atrial depolarization, it WILL put
out the ventricular spike.

*Adding R on the end indicates a rate
responsive function in the pacemaker; i.e.
VVIR, DDDR. e.g. If patient exercises the
PPM will ↑ the intrinsic set rate

- -

POOR MAN'S 12-LEAD ECG

If monitoring w/ 3-leads:
- Monitor in I
- Move the white electrode to the black electrode position and the black electrode to the V1 (MCL_1) position
- Black lead now becomes MCL_1 to MCL_6 (V1 – V6) by physically moving the electrode around the precordium

OR

- Monitor in III
- Move the red electrode to the V1 (MCL_1) position
- Red lead now becomes MCL_1 to MCL_6 (V1 – V6) by physically moving the electrode around the precordium

*By printing off a strip each time the electrodes are moved, a 9-Lead ECG can be obtained – the augmented leads will be missing.

- -

PULSE PRESSURE

Difference between the systolic blood pressure and the diastolic blood pressure

WNL: 25 – 40 mmHg

If ↑ consider:
- Thyrotoxicosis
- AV Fistula
- Patent Ductus Arteriosis
- Aortic Insufficiency
- Late Shock

If ↓ consider:
- Pericarditis
- Pericardial Effusion
- Pericardial Tamponade
- Aortic Stenosis
- Tachycardia
- Early Shock

- -

QT INTERVAL – RATE ADJUSTED

HR	QTc	HR	QTc
40	0.48	85	0.33
45	0.43	90	0.32
50	0.41	95	0.31
55	0.40	100	0.30
60	0.38	110	0.30
65	0.37	120	0.29
70	0.36	130	0.28
75	0.35	140	0.26
80	0.34	150	0.25

↑ QT: Hypocalcemia, hypokalemia, hypomagnesemia, AMI, TCA, quinidine, procainamide, myocarditis, CHF, MVP

↓ QT: Hypercalcemia, hyperkalemia, digoxin

- - - - - - - - - - - - - - - - - - - -

REENTRY PATHWAYS

Wolff-Parkinson White (WPW):

- Preexcitation syndrome occurring from Kent bundles that directly link the atria to the ventricles thus bypassing the AV node and infranodal system. A short PR interval is seen along w/ a delta wave on ECG.
    - Type A: In V1 there is a positive initial deflection and a dominant R-wave is seen. Q-waves may be seen in II, III, aVF
    *May mimic a posterior wall MI

34

- Type B: In V1 there is a negative initial deflection and an rS or QS complex is seen
  *May mimic an inferior wall MI

- Type C: In V1 there is a positive delta wave and in V5 and/or V6 there is a negative or isoelectric delta wave

*If the impulse is directed down the normal AV conducting pathway and up the bypass tract (orthodromic tachycardia) the QRS complex will be normal and the delta wave will NOT be seen which is usually the case of reentrant SVT

*If the impulse is directed down the bypass tract and retrograde through the AV node (antidromic tachycardia) the QRS complex will be wide and the delta wave should be visible

*Treatment differs
- If narrow QRS complex administer adenosine or verapamil
- If wide QRS complex the patient is at risk for VF, therefore treat w/ procainamide or cardioversion
  *β-blockers and Ca^{++} channel blockers should be avoided

(con't)

Reentry Pathways – WPW (con't)

-    If WPW w/ atrial fibrillation or atrial flutter
     w/ rapid ventricular response, use
     cardioversion, procainamide or lidocaine
     *Digoxin should be avoided since it can
     shorten the refractory period and
     enhance bypass tract conduction

Lown-Ganong-Levine Syndrome (LGL):

-    Preexcitation syndrome occurring from
     James fibers which are a continuation of
     the posterior internodal tract. These
     fibers abnormally connect the atria
     muscle to HIS bundle. A short PR
     interval is seen with a normal QRS.

Mahaim Fibers:

-    Preexcitation syndrome occurring from
     conductive tracts of myogenic tissue that
     originate from the AV node, HIS bundle
     or bundle branches and abnormally insert
     into the ventricular septum. All or part of
     the infranodal conducting system is
     bypassed after the impulse travels
     normally through the AV node. A normal
     PR interval is seen along w/ a delta
     wave.

- -

SWAN-GANZ CATHETER READINGS

CVP/RAP (proximal port): 1 – 6 mmHg
- Central Venous Pressure/Right Atrial Pressure evaluates the patient's volume status
- Helps in identifying shock type
- Reflects RV preload – RVEDP
    - ↑: Cardiogenic shock, RV failure/infarct, volume overload, pulmonary HTN/vasoconstriction, cardiac tamponade, constrictive pericarditis, tricuspid valve stenosis/regurgitation, PEEP

    - ↓: Hypovolemic shock – absolute or relative, septic shock

Interpretation of CVP Waveform

a-wave: R atrial contraction
- ↑: Pulmonary HTN, pulmonary embolus, tricuspid stenosis, cor pulmonale

- ↓: Atrial fibrillation
    - Cannon a-waves: 3° AVB and AV dissociation (irregular cannon a-waves), junctional tachycardia (regular cannon a-waves)

(con't)

Swan-Ganz – Interpret CVP Wave (con't)
x-descent: R atrial relaxation

c-wave: On x-descent, caused from upward
displacement of the tricuspid valve
during early systole

v-wave: R atrial filling against closed tricuspid
valve, occurs just prior to carotid
pulse

- ↑: In conditions causing ↑ a-waves and
in tricuspid regurgitation

y-descent: R atrial pressure ↓ due to filling of
RV after tricuspid valve opens

- Prolonged: Tricuspid stenosis

RVP (during insertion): $\dfrac{15 - 30 \text{ mmHg}}{0 - 8 \text{ mmHg}}$

*Right Ventricular Pressure

PAP (distal port): $\dfrac{15 - 30 \text{ mmHg}}{4 - 12 \text{ mmHg}}$

Mean: 10 – 20 mmHg

*Pulmonary Arterial Pressure

38

- ↑: Cardiogenic shock, COPD, pulmonary HTN, pulmonary embolus, mitral regurgitation, mitral stenosis, aortic stenosis, aortic regurgitation, ASD, VSD, PEEP, volume overload

- ↓: Septic shock, hypovolemic shock

PCWP/LAP (during wedging): 4 – 12 mmHg
- Pulmonary Capillary Wedge Pressure/ Left Atrial Pressure reflects LA and LV pressure
- Measure at end-expiration from phlebostatic axis w/ HOB < 30°
- ∅ leave balloon inflated for > 15 sec

  - ↑: Cardiogenic shock, COPD, pulmonary HTN, pulmonary embolus, mitral regurgitation, mitral stenosis, aortic stenosis, pulmonary edema, PEEP, volume overload

  - ↓: Hypovolemic shock – relative or absolute, septic shock, neurogenic shock, non-cardiac pulmonary edema

*Pulmonary congestion = PCWP ≥ 18 mmHg
*Pulmonary edema = PCWP ≥ 25 mmHg

(con't)

Swan-Ganz (con't)

CO: 4 – 8 L/min
- Cardiac output determines shock extent, LV function, patient status
  - ↑: Neurogenic shock, septic shock

  - ↓: Cardiogenic shock, hypovolemic shock – relative or absolute, late septic shock

CI: 2.5 – 4.5 $L/min/m^2$
- Cardiac index is the measurement of the CO/m^2 of BSA
- CO/BSA
  - ↑: Vasogenic shock

  - ↓: Hypovolemic shock, cardiogenic shock, vasogenic shock

* < 3.0 = inadequate CO
* < 1.8 = cardiogenic shock

RVEF: 46 – 50%
- Proportion of blood ejected during each ventricular contraction compared w/ the total ventricular volume
- Index of ventricular function
- RVEDV normal is 80 – 150 ml/m^2
- $\frac{SV}{RVEDV}$, where RVEDV = SV/RVEF

SVI: 40 – 70 ml/beat/m^2
- Stroke Volume Index = $\dfrac{CI}{HR}$

SVR: 900 – 1200 dynes·sec·m^2/cm^5
- Systemic Vascular Resistance

- $\dfrac{MAP - RAP}{CO} \times 80$

PVR: 200 – 400 dynes·sec·m^2/cm^5
- Pulmonary Vascular Resistance
- $\dfrac{(PAP - PCWP)}{CO} \times 80$

RVSWI: 4 – 8 g·m/m^2
- RV Stroke Work Index – work needed to move the stroke volume across the pulmonary circulation into the left heart
- (PAP – CVP) × SVI × 0.0136

LVSWI: 40 – 60 g·m/m^2
- LV Stroke Work Index – work needed to move the stroke volume into the aorta
- (MAP – PCWP) × SVI × 0.0136

(con't)

Swan-Ganz (con't)

SVO_2: 65 – 75%

- Mixed venous O_2
- Indicative of the balance between oxygen delivery and oxygen consumption
- 5% variation for > 10 min indicates a significant change
- $SaO_2 - (Vo_2/Q \times Hgb)$

  ↓: Hypoxia, ARDS, hypovolemia, ↓ Hgb, fever, MI, CHF, shivering, thyrotoxicosis, MI

  ↑: Permanently wedged catheter, sepsis, burns, hepatitis, pancreatitis, left-to-right shunts, CO poisoning, CN toxicity, inotropic excess

- - - - - - - - - - - - - - - - - - - -

THROMBOLYTIC THERAPY CHECKLIST – ACUTE MYOCARDIAL INFARCTION

Absolute Contraindication

- Previous hemorrhagic stroke @ any time; other strokes or cerebrovascular events within 1 year
- Known intracranial neoplasm
- Active internal bleeding (except menses)
- Suspected aortic dissection

Cautions: Relative Contraindications

- Severe uncontrolled HTN @ presentation (BP > 180/110)
- Other intracerebral pathology
- Current use of anticoagulants (INR > 2 – 3), known bleeding diathesis
- Recent trauma (2 – 4 weeks), including head trauma
- Prolonged (> 10 min) and potentially traumatic CPR
- Major surgery (< 3 weeks prior)
- Noncompressible vascular punctures
- Recent (2 – 4 weeks) internal bleeding
- For streptokinase/anistreplase: prior exposure (especially in previous 2 years); prior allergic reaction to streptokinase
- Pregnancy
- Active peptic ulcer
- History of chronic severe HTN

TORSADES DE POINTES

Causes:

- Class 1a: disopyramide, quinidine, procainamide, amiodarone
- Class 3: amiodarone
- Phenothiazines
- TCA's
- Hypokalemia
- Hypomagnesemia
- Hypocalcemia
- Erythromycin w/ astemazole
- Ketoconazole w/ astemazole

Tx:

- $MgSO_4$ 1 – 2 g bolus over 1 – 2 min followed by 1 – 2 g over 1 hr
  *Up to 4 – 6 g may be required to suppress Torsades de Pointes
  *SE: Short-lasting flushing, mild hypotension
- Overdrive pacing (TCP or TVP) up to 180 beats per minute
- Isoproterenol infusion 2 – 8 µg/min
- Cardioversion/defibrillation

VT – QUICK GUIDE TO EVALUATE BROAD COMPLEX TACHYCARDIA

Look at lead V1, if QRS pattern is mainly (+), the following favor VT:

- Monophasic or biphasic QRS
- R to S ratio < 1 (deep S-wave) in V6
- L rabbit ear taller than R in V1

Look at lead V1 – V2, if QRS pattern is mainly (−), the following favor VT:

- Broad R-wave (> 0.03 sec)
- Slurred/notched downslope of S-wave
- > 0.06 sec from R-wave to nadir of S-wave

Look at V6, if there is any Q-wave in presence of (−) deflection in V1, 98% accuracy for VT

Look at Lead 1, should be (+), if (−) high suspicion for VT

*Diagnostic: Fusion beats and/or capture beats

*Suggestive:
- Extreme RAD (− 90 to − 180°)
- QRS complexes are all (−) or all (+) in V1 – V6
- AV dissociation

- -

WELLEN'S SYNDROME
Warns of critical LAD stenosis

Criteria:
- Prior angina
- Enzyme increase < 4%
- No pathological Q-wave
- No loss of R-wave progression
- Little or no ST-segment elevation
- Progressive T-wave inversion from previous ECG's
- Deeply inverted symmetrical T-waves
- Found in V2 – V3

*Patient should be taken to the cardiac catheterization lab for evaluation as soon as feasible

- -

FORMULAS

ALVEOLAR-ARTERIAL OXYGEN GRADIENT

$(760 - 47) \times 0.21 - 1.2(PaCO_2) - PaO_2$

*Normal is 10 – 20 mmHg
*See full explanation in the pulmonary text under same heading

----

ANION GAP

$Na^+ - (Cl^- + HCO_3^-) = 8$ to 12 mEq/L

Elevated gap may be due to:
- DKA
- Alcohol
- Renal failure
- Lactic acidosis
- INH
- No food (starvation)
- Generalized sz
- Sepsis
- ASA
- Rhabdomyolysis
- Ethylene glycol
- Iron
- Methanol
- Paraldehyde

*DARLINGS ARE IMPortant
*Check serum osmolarity gap

(con't)

Anion Gap (con't)

*Must correct the serum HCO_3^-:

Corrected HCO_3^- = excess anion gap + measured HCO_3^-

- Corrected HCO_3^- wnl: then any ↓ in the measured HCO_3^- is due to the anion gap acidosis
- Corrected HCO_3^- ↑: there is an underlying metabolic alkalosis
- Corrected HCO_3^- ↓: there is an underlying nongap acidosis

*Excess anion gap =

measured anion gap – wnl anion gap

*Use 12 for wnl anion gap

Decreased gap may be due to:
- ↑ K^+, Mg^{++}, Li^{++} ingestion
- multiple myeloma
- ↓ albumin
- nephrotic syndrome

Normal gap may be due to:
- intestinal loss – diarrhea, pancreatic fistula, biliary drainage
- carbonic anhydrase inhibitors
- renal tubular acidosis
- mineralocorticoid deficiency
- exogenous Cl^- or K^+ administration

*Differential diagnosis of hyperchloremic metabolic acidosis can be obtained by obtaining the urinary anion gap along w/ the urinary pH:

Anion Gap (Urine) = $(U_{Na} + U_K - U_{Cl})$
- (−) gap indicates loss of GI HCO_3
- (+) gap indicates altered distal urinary tract acidification
- ↓ urinary pH w/ ↑ serum K^+ and (+) gap indicates aldosterone insufficiency
- Urinary pH > 5.5 w/ ↑ serum K^+ indicates hyperkalemic distal renal tubular acidosis
- Urinary pH > 5.5 w/ wnl or ↓ serum K^+ indicates renal tubular acidosis

----

BASE DEFICIT – NaHCO$_3$ DOSE
mmol of base needed to correct the pH of 1 liter whole blood to a pH of 7.40

Mild   2 – 5 mmol/L
Moderate 6 – 14 mmol/L
Severe   > 15 mmol/L

Base deficit $\times$ kg wt $\times$ 0.3 = dose of NaHCO$_3$*
*Administer ¼ to ½ of the calculated dose

OR

(Desired NaHCO$_3$ – actual NaHCO$_3$) $\times$ 0.5 $\times$ kg wt = mEq NaHCO$_3$ to be administered over 30 min
*Desired NaHCO$_3$ level is 15 – 20 mEq/L

(con't)

49

Base Deficit (con't)

NOTE: 2.5 mEq/L NaHCO₃ × kg wt, infused over ½ hr, will ↑ the serum bicarbonate level by 5 mEq/L

*Base deficit = ongoing ischemia

BODY SURFACE AREA

Square root of: $\dfrac{kg\ wt \times cm\ ht}{3600}$

COLLOID ONCOTIC PRESSURE

COP = 2.1 × serum total protein

WNL: 17 – 25 in the supine patient
22 – 29 in the upright patient

*If using Hetastarch or Dextran, the COP must be measured, or else, the calculated COP will be falsely lowered

----

CONVERSION FORMULAS

Length
- 1 in = 2.54 cm
- 1 cm = 0.39 in

Liquid
- 1 fluid oz ≈ 30 ml
- 1 Tbs = 15 ml
- 1 tsp = 5 ml

Temperature
- $°C = (°F - 32) ÷ 1.8$
- $°F = (°C \times 1.8) + 32$

Weight
- 1 lb = 0.45 kg
- 1 kg = 2.2 lb
- 10 grains = 650 mg
- 400 µg = 1/150 grain

CREATININE CLEARANCE

$$\frac{\text{Urine Cr (mg/100ml)} \times \text{Urine volume (ml)}}{\text{Serum Cr (mg/100ml)} \times \text{time (use 1440 min)}}$$

*Males: 100 – 125 ml/min
*Females: 85 – 105 ml/min

*Obtain 24 hr urine when creatinine is stable

DEGREE OF DEHYDRATION

$$\frac{\text{pre-illness wt} - \text{illness wt}}{\text{illness wt}} = \% \text{ dehydration}$$

Infants	Children	S/S
5% (50 ml/kg)	3% (30 ml/kg)	Slight ↑ HR, slightly dry mucosa, concentrated urine
10% (100 ml/kg)	6% (60 ml/kg)	↑ HR, dry mucosa, ↓ skin turgor, oliguria, sunken anterior fontanel
15% (150 ml/kg)	9% (90 ml/kg)	↓ BP, delayed capillary refill, Kussmaul breathing, obtunded

----

ET TUBE SIZE

$$\text{ETT Size} = \frac{16 + \text{age (yrs)}}{4}$$

*Use an **uncuffed** tube in children under 6 yo
*Cuff pressure 10 – 20 cm H_2O
***Depth of Insertion in cm** = (Age ÷ 2) + 12

FRACTIONAL EXCRETION OF Na⁺

$$FENa = \frac{(Urine\ Na) \times (Plasma\ Cr)}{(Urine\ Cr) \times (Plasma\ Na)} \times 100$$

*Prerenal azotemia if FENa < 1%
- $U_{osm} > 500$
- $U_{Na} < 20$ mEq/L
- UA = normal

*ATN if FENa > 2%
- $U_{osm} < 350$
- $U_{Na} > 40$ mEq/L
- UA = granular casts

Causes of ARF: aminoglycosides, gentamycin, ACE inhibitors, NSAIDS, IVP dye, emboli, rhabdomyolysis

---

FREE WATER DEFICIT

Free H_2O deficit =
$$\frac{0.6 \times kg\ wt \times (serum\ Na^+ - 140)}{140}$$

*Averages 4 ml/kg for q mEq that serum Na⁺ exceeds 145 mEq/L

GLOMERULAR FILTRATION RATE

Estimated: $\dfrac{(140 - \text{age in yrs}) \times \text{kg wt}}{72 \times \text{serum creatinine}}$

Measured: $\dfrac{\text{Cr Clearance} + \text{Urea Clearance}}{2}$

*For female multiply by 0.85
*Normal young adult has a creatinine
 clearance of 80 – 125 ml/min
*If creatinine clearance = 30 ml/min, give 1/3
 of the adult dose of the medication . If 25
 ml/min, give ¼ of the adult dose, etc.

HYDRATION / CALORIES METABOLIZED / ELECTROLYTES / FLUID LOSS / CALCULATION FOR MAINTENANCE IV FLUIDS

Quick Method
4 ml/kg for each kg from 0 to 10 +
2 ml/kg for each kg from 10 to 20 +
1 ml/kg for each kg > 20
*This will calculate an hourly rate
*NOT suitable for neonates < 14 d

24 Hour Method

100 ml/kg for each kg from 0 to 10 +
50 ml/kg for each kg from 10 to 20 +
20 ml/kg for each kg > 20 for a 24 hr period

*If febrile add 12% for each degree > 37.8°
 rectally
*Add 20 mEq KCl/L if no renal or adrenal
 insufficiency
*NOT suitable for neonates < 14 d

Use: $D_5$0.2 NS if patient < 10 kg
     $D_5$0.33 NS if patient between 10 – 20 kg
     $D_5$0.45 NS if patient > 20 kg

Calories Metabolized

*Use the 24 Hour method formula using Cal in
place of ml and substitute 10 Cal/kg for each
kg > 20

Electrolytes

Na^+ 3 mEq/100 ml H_2O metabolized
Cl^- 2 mEq/100 ml H_2O metabolized
K^+ 2 mEq/100 ml H_2O metabolized

Losses

Urine 65 ml/100 ml H_2O metabolized
* < 10 ml/100 ml H_2O metabolized = oliguria
Skin 30 ml/100 ml H_2O metabolized
Lungs 15 ml/100 ml H_2O metabolized
Stool 5 ml/100 ml H_2O metabolized

IDEAL BODY WEIGHT

Male: 106# up to 5 ft, then 6# for q inch
Female: 100# up to 5 ft, then 5# for q inch

*If the patient is obese, subtract the patient's
 calculated IBW from the true weight and add
 the difference to the calculated IBW

Broca's Index

IBW in kg = (ht in cm − 100)
*1 ft = 30 cm

*25 − 100% of IBW = Obese
 > 100% of IBW = Morbidly Obese

INTRAVENOUS MEDICATION RATE/DOSE

To find rate: $RATE = \dfrac{DOSE \times KG\ WT \times 60}{CONC}$

To find dose: $DOSE = \dfrac{(CONC\ /\ 60) \times RATE}{KG\ WT}$

OSMOLARITY – SERUM

$2(Na^+) + (glucose/18) + (BUN/2.8)$

*Normal serum osmolarity is 280 – 295
*Osmolal Gap: if the measured minus the
            calculated gap is > 10 look for
            ethanol, methanol, ethylene
            glycol, isopropanol or some
            other unidentified toxin
*If patient ingested ethanol, divide the level by
4.6; if methanol, divide the level by 3.2; if
ethylene-glycol, divide the level by 6.2; and if
isopropanol, divide the level by 6

OXYGENATION

$PaO_2 \div FiO_2$

< 200 = ARDS
< 300 = acute lung injury

*Every 10% ↑ in FiO_2, ↑ PaO_2 by 50 – 60 torr

OXYGEN CONTENT

$(Hgb \times 1.34 \times SaO_2) + (0.003 \times PaO_2)$

*Each g of Hgb will bind 1.34 ml O_2 when fully
 saturated w/ oxygen
*Oxygen saturation must be in the form of a
 decimal
*Can use 75% oxygen saturation to calculate
 the oxygen content in mixed venous blood

*For a Hgb = 15 g/dl, SaO_2 = 0.98 and PaO_2 =
 100 mmHg, the O_2 content should be 20
 ml/100 ml (200 ml/L)

OXYGEN DELIVERY

$Do_2 = Q \times 13.4 \times Hgb \times SaO_2$

WNL: 520 – 570 ml/min/m^2
*Q = flow = cardiac output
*Calculates the rate of O_2 transport in arterial
 blood

OXYGEN EXTRACTION RATIO

$$O_2ER = (SaO_2 - Svo_2/SaO_2) \times 100$$

WNL: 20 – 30% (0.2 – 0.3)
*O_2 deficit if > 0.5 – only applies if O_2 delivery is impaired
*Calculates the fractional uptake of O_2 into the tissues

When $SaO_2 - Svo_2$ is:
20 – 30%	Normal
30 – 50%	↓ CO, anemia, hypermetabolism, hypovolemia
> 50 – 60%	Hypovolemic shock, high risk of dysoxia – think of transfusing the patient

---

OXYGENATION INDEX

$$OI = \frac{P_{aw} \times FiO_2 \times 100}{PaO_2 \text{ (post ductal)}}$$

- Oxygenation Index (OI) > 40 predicts a mortality > 90%
- OI 25 – 40 = mortality of 50 – 80%

OXYGEN UPTAKE

$$Vo_2 = Q \times 13.4 \times Hgb \times (SaO_2 - Svo_2)$$

WNL: $110 - 160$ ml/min/m^2
*Q = flow = cardiac output
*Calculates the O_2 consumption from the tissues
*The calculated Vo_2 must Δ by 15% to be considered significant while the measured only needs to Δ by 5%

To correct Vo_2:
- ↑ CVP to $10 - 12$ mmHg or PCWP to $18 - 20$ mmHg w/ fluids
- If CO ↓ and CVP or PCWP is not, ↑ CVP or PCWP as stated above
- If CO ↓ and CVP or PCWP ↑, start dobutamine @ 3 µg/kg/min and titrate to obtain a CI > 3.0 L/min/m^2
  *If ↓ BP, start dopamine @ 5 µg/kg/min
- If Vo_2 < 100 ml/min/m^2, use volume to obtain a CVP $8 - 10$ mmHg or PCWP $18 - 20$ mmHg along w/ inotropes to achieve a CI > 4.5 L/min/m^2
  *Correct anemia if Hgb < 8.0 g/dl

- If $Vo_2 > 100$ ml/min/m^2 and lactic acid level > 4 mmol/L w/ s/s shock, ↓ the patient's metabolic rate by using sedation w/ or w/o paralytics and/or stopping feedings and/or providing grouped patient care i.e. baths, visits, etc all timed together until the $Vo_2 > 160$ ml/min/m^2
- If lactic acid level < 4 mmol/L, observe the patient

PNEUMOTHORAX PERCENTAGE

$$1 - \frac{\text{distance from midline to lung parenchyma}}{\text{distance from midline to thoracic wall}}$$

RULE OF 6

$n \times 6 \times$ kg wt = mg to add to 100 ml of fluid
*1 ml/hr = n µg/kg/min

n = Drug concentration

*n = 0.1 for isoproterenol, epinephrine, norepinephrine
*n = 0.3 for prostaglandin
*n = 1 for dopamine, dobutamine, nitroprusside
*n = 10 for lidocaine

SHOCK INDEX (SI)

$SI = HR \div SBP$

WNL: $0.5 - 0.7$

If > 0.9 it indicates:
- $\downarrow$ systemic oxygenation
- $\downarrow$ LV stroke work (i.e. stroke index)
- $\downarrow$ cardiac function
- Global ischemia

SHUNT EQUATION

R$\rightarrow$L Shunt on FiO_2 1.0: $\dfrac{Qs}{Qt} = \dfrac{(A-aDO_2)}{20}$

WNL: < 10

URINARY PROTEIN EXCRETION

$U_{Pr} \div U_{Cr}$

WNL: < 0.2 (200 mg/d)
Glomerular Disease = > 3.5

*Done as spot check; as accurate as 24 hr UA
*Δ in urinary concentration does not Δ ratio

- -

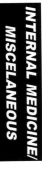

INTERNAL MEDICINE/
MISCELANEOUS

BLOOD AND COMPONENT THERAPY

PRBC

Use:

- Evidence of impaired tissue oxygenation
- Ongoing coronary or cerebrovascular ischemia in patients w/ normovolemia
- $O_{2ER} > 0.5$ (if CO is adequate)
- To correct Hgb < 7 g/dl if the patient is at risk for myocardial ischemia/infarction, cerebral ischemia/infarction or cardiac dysfunction

Dose: 3 – 4 ml/kg

  *1u PRBC = 250 – 300 ml which will $\uparrow$ Hgb 1 g/dl and $\uparrow$ Hct by 3%

  *$\uparrow$ Vo_2 after transfusion of one unit PRBC indicates a beneficial response

Volume of PRBC (mL) =

$$EBV (ml) \times \frac{Desired\ Hct - Actual\ Hct}{Hct\ of\ PRBC's}$$

*EBV Adult: 75 ml/kg
*Hct of PRBC's: 55 – 70%

Reticulocyte Index

Retic Count $\times$ (Hct/45) $\times$ 100

WNL: 1 – 2
*If $\uparrow$ = bone marrow functioning   (con't)

63

Blood & Component Rx (con't)
Platelets
Use: Active bleeding
- platelet count < 50,000/mm^3 not associated w/ an immune mechanism
- platelet count > 50,000/mm^3 associated w/ a condition that causes platelet dysfunction i.e. cardiopulmonary bypass

Use: Prophylaxis
- platelet count < 5,000/mm^3
- platelet count < 20,000/mm^3 in a patient with a high bleeding risk
- platelet count < 50,000/mm^3 in a patient with a planned endoscopic bx, lumbar puncture, major surgery or recent surgery

Dose: 10 ml/kg
*1 U platelets ↑ count by 5,000 to 10,000/mm^3
*Goal is a platelet count of 50,000/mm^3
*Pooled platelets = 6 – 12 U condensed to 1 U. Use for volume restriction.

Fresh Frozen Plasma
Use: Deficiency of plasma proteins
associated w/ liver dz, DIC, vitamin K
deficiency, warfarin overdose

Dose: Start w/ 4 U FFP

Use: Hypofibrinogenemia
*Normal levels:
Adult 200 – 400 mg/dl
Child: 250 mg/dl
Premature Infant: 150 – 200 mg/dl

Dose: 10 – 15 ml/kg FFP q 12 – 24 hr w/
1 – 2 bags of cryoprecipitate/5 kg

Use: Single factor deficiency

*To determine the number of units of factor to
administer:
1. kg wt × 70 ml = blood volume in ml
2. blood volume × (1 – Hct) = plasma
volume
3. plasma volume × (desired factor
level – initial factor level) = U of factor
to infuse
*1 U factor = 1 U FFP
*30% factor activity is usually sufficient for
hemostasis

(con't)

Blood & Component Rx (con't)
Cryoprecipitate
Use: DIC, fibrinogen deficiency, severe liver
       dz, dilutional hypofibrinogenemia

Dose: see formula above in FFP

*Each 10 – 15 ml unit (bag) contains 80 U of
factor VIII, at least 150 mg of fibrinogen,
along w/ von Willebrand factor and
fibronectin

Use: factor VIII deficiency

Dose: 1 – 2 U cryoprecipitate/5 kg q 8 – 12 hr
*Goal is to ↑ the factor VIII activity to
 between 80% and 100%
- -

DIABETIC KETOACIDOSIS, ADULT

Dx:
- Glucose > 300 mg/dl
- Metabolic acidosis per ABG
    - PH < 7.30
    - HCO_3 < 15 mEq/L
- Ketonemia
- Ketonuria

*Obtain electrolytes, BUN, Cr, glucose, CBC, ABG, UA
*If ketone/fruity breath expect pH to be < 7.12

Tx: Adult:
- Regular insulin 0.33 U/kg bolus
- Insulin gtt @ 0.1 U/kg/hr
    *Mix 100 U/1000ml NS
    (10 ml/hr = 1 U/hr)
- 1 – 2 liters NS over 1 hr, then 150 – 200 ml/hr
- If K^+ low or wnl, administer 20 – 30 mEq/hr PRN to maintain wnl serum K^+. Start after first 1000 ml fluid.
    *K^+ deficit is usually 8 – 10 mEq/kg
- If K^+ high – hold KCl until adequate UO, then add KCl @ 20 mEq/hr
- If pH < 7.1 consider administering $NaHCO_3$ 50 mEq over 1 – 2 hr

(con't)

Diabetic Ketoacidosis (con't)

*This therapy should lower serum glucose by 75 – 100 mg/dl/hr

- Obtain serum glucose q 1 hr
- If glucose falls faster, continue insulin gtt and add D_5W to IV fluid
- If glucose falls < 50 mg/dl/hr, increase insulin to 0.14 – 0.2 U/kg/hr

*HPO_4, which is depleted in DKA, will drop w/ insulin therapy. PO_4 improves release of O_2 to tissues. Therefore, replace PRN and consider replacing K^+ as ½ KCl and ½ KPO_4 for the first 8 hr, then all as KCl after 8 hr.
*Excessive PO_4 may induce hypocalcemic tetany

- When serum glucose < 300 mg/dl, add D_5W and continue insulin gtt @ 0.1 U/kg/hr
- When serum glucose < 250 mg/dl and the patient is NOT spilling ketones in urine, discontinue insulin gtt 1 – 2 hr after administration of SQ insulin
- Start regular insulin 0.25 U/kg SQ q 4 – 8 hr
- Obtain serum glucose q 6 hr and PRN

- -

ELECTROLYTE DISTURBANCES, ADULT

Hypocalcemia: Serum Ca^{++} < 8.5 mg/dl or ionized Ca^{++} < 4.40 mg/dl
Circumoral paresthesias, paresthesias of the digits, sz, Chovstek's sign, Trousseau's sign

Causes: Hypoparathyroidism, pseudohypoparathyroidism, vitamin D deficiency, renal failure, magnesium deficiency, multiple blood transfusions

*If the patient has hypoalbuminemia, adjust the Ca^{++} level as follows:

Adjusted Ca^{**} =
Serum Ca^{++} + 0.8 × (4 – albumin)
Tx: Adult: Ca^{++} gluconate:
- 5 – 15 g/d IV/PO ÷ q 6 hr

Hypercalcemia: Serum Ca^{++} > 10.5 mg/dl or ionized Ca^{++} < 5.4 mg/dl
Anorexia, N/V, constipation, muscle weakness, polyuria, polydipsia, neurotic behavior, dysrhythmias

(con't)

Electrolyte Disturbances (con't)
Causes: Hyperparathyroidism, ectopic PTH-
producing tumors, vitamin D excess,
malignancy, immobilization

Tx: Adult:

- Vigorous IV hydration w/ NS
- Furosemide 40 – 80 mg IV q
  2 – 6 hr
  *Can be added to NS to
  maintain UO 100 – 200 ml/hr
- Calcitonin 4 U/kg IV first dose,
  then 4 U/kg IM/SQ q 12 hr
  *Skin test for allergy before
  administration
- Hydrocortisone 200 mg IV/d ÷
  q 8 – 12 hr
- Etidronate disodium 7.5
  mg/kg/d mixed in 250 ml NS
  and infused over 2 hr if
  unresponsive to above
  measures
  *Given for 1 – 4 consecutive
  days

Hypokalemia: Serum K^+ < 3.5 mEq/L
Anorexia, N/V, fatigue, muscle
weakness, ↓ bowel motility,
dysrhythmias, paresthesias,
flat T-waves on ECG, MAT

Causes: Renovascular dz, excess renin, excess mineralocorticoid, Cushing's syndrome, renal tubular acidosis, antibiotics, diuretics, cystic fibrosis, skin losses, GI losses, alkalosis, excessive insulin, leukemia

Tx: Adult: 10 – 15 mEq KCl/hr IV

Sliding Scale:
3.6 – 3.9   20 mEq IV/PO
3.5 – 3.2   40 mEq IV/PO
3.1 – 2.8   50 mEq IV/PO
< 2.8   Call Physician

Hyperkalemia: Serum K^+ > 5.8 mEq/L
Dysrhythmias, bradycardia, muscle weakness, flaccid paralysis, tall tented T-waves on ECG

Causes: Cell breakdown, congenital adrenal hypoplasia, renal failure, hemolysis, hypoaldosteronism, aldosterone insensitivity, low insulin, K^+-sparing diuretics, leukocytosis, metabolic acidosis, thrombocytosis

(con't)

Electrolyte Dist – Hyperkalemia (con't)
Tx: Adult:

- 10% Ca^{++}(gluconate or Cl)
  1 g IV over 10 – 20 min
  ***∅ give if patient taking
  digoxin – assume digoxin
  toxicity as cause of
  hyperkalemia**
  *CaCl more readily available
  once administered
- $D_{50}W$ 50 ml IV
- Regular insulin 5 – 10 U IV
- Can give 1000 ml $D_{20}W$ w/
  40 – 80 U regular insulin over
  the next 2 – 4 hr
- $NaHCO_3$ 50 mEq IV over
  10 – 20 min
- Kayexalate 15 – 25 g w/ 50 ml
  20% sorbitol PO q 4 – 6 hr
  OR
- Kayexalate 20 g in 200 ml of a
  20% sorbitol solution PR q 4 hr
  *1 g Kayexalate eliminates
  1 mEq K^+
- Emergent dialysis PRN

Hypomagnesemia: Serum Mg^{++} < 1.5 mEq/L
Dysrhythmias,
neuromuscular irritability,
disorientation

Causes: Furosemide, aminoglycosides,
digitalis, diarrhea, alcohol abuse,
DM, acute MI

Tx: Adult: 25 – 50 mg/kg q 4 – 6 hr × 3 – 4
doses

Hypermagnesemia: Serum Mg^{++} > 2.5 mEq/L
Hypotension, flushing,
drowsiness, ↓ DTR's,
respiratory depression,
coma, cardiac arrest

Causes: Impaired renal function

Tx: Adult:
- Hemodialysis
- Ca^{++} gluconate 1 g IV over
  2 – 3 min
- If patient can tolerate fluids,
  aggressive fluid administration
  w/ furosemide may be effective

(con't)

Electrolyte Disturbances (con't)

Hyponatremia: Serum Na^+ < 135 mEq/L
Anorexia, N/V, confusion,
lethargy, muscle cramps,
muscular twitching, sz,
papilledema

Causes: GI loss, third spacing, skin loss,
nephrotic syndrome, CHF, SIADH,
factitious

(desired Na^+ – actual Na^+) $\times$ 0.6 $\times$ kg wt =
mEq Na^+ to replace

Volume of 3% NaCl = $\dfrac{mEq\ Na^+\ needed}{0.513\ mEq\ Na/ml}$

Tx:
- Slow infusion: 15 ml/hr
  *Use if the patient has a slow rise in Na^+

- Rapid infusion: 1.0 – 1.5 ml/kg/hr
  *Administer for 2 – 3 hr
  *Risk of sz, coma, central pontine
  myelinolysis

*NOTE: $\varnothing$ correct faster than 8 – 12 mEq/d
(0.3 – 0.5 mEq/L/hr) due to risk of
central pontine myelinolysis

*Add $NaHCO_3$ as needed for acidosis
*Add 20 – 40 mEq KCl/L after adequate UO
*Hyperglycemia:

- $Na^+ \downarrow$ by 1.6 mEq/L for q 100 mg/dl $\uparrow$ in glucose

*Hyperproteinemia:

- $Na^+ \downarrow$ by $0.25 \times$ [protein (g/dl) – 8]

*Hyperlipidemia:

- $Na^+ \downarrow$ $0.002 \times$ lipid (mg/dl)

Hypernatremia: Serum $Na^+ > 145$ mEq/L
Thirst, $\uparrow$ temperature, edematous dry tongue, tenacious sputum, hallucinations, lethargy, irritability, focal or grand mal sz, hyperreflexia

Causes: $\downarrow$ free H_2O intake, GI loss, skin loss, diuretics, nephropathy, diabetes insipidus, excess Na^+ administration, mineralocorticoid excess

$$H_2O \text{ deficit} = \frac{\text{serum } Na^+ - 140}{140} \times 0.6 \times \text{kg wt}$$

(con't)

Electrolyte Dist – Hypernatremia (con't)

Tx:

- If hypovolemic replace volume first w/ NS or LR until BP and tissue perfusion are adequate
- Next, use $D_50.45$ NaCl
- If Na^+ ↓ too quickly, Δ to $D_50.33$ NaCl or $D_50.2$ NaCl – **usually used in children**
- Add Ca^{++} as needed

*NOTE: Ø correct faster than 10 – 15 mEq/L/d (0.5 mEq/L/hr) due to risk of cerebral edema, sz, pulmonary edema and death

*Each liter of H_2O deficit raises the serum Na^+ by 3 – 5 mEq/L
*Add 20 – 40 mEq KCl/L which aids water entry into the cells
*Replace total fluid deficit over 48 – 72 hrs

Hypophosphatemia: Serum PO_4 < 3.0 mg/dl Muscle weakness, pain and tenderness, mental status Δ's, respiratory failure, paresthesias, cardiomyopathy

Causes: Phosphate binding antacids, renal tubular phosphate reabsorption defects, movement of PO_4 into cells

76

Tx: Adult:

     Mild: 2.0 – 2.5
- 0.0125 mM/kg/hr IV × 6 hrs

     Moderate: 0.5 – 2.0
- 0.04 mM/kg/hr IV × 6 hrs
  OR
- 0.06 mM/kg/hr IV × 4 hrs

     Severe: < 0.5
- 0.125 mM/kg/hr IV × 4 hrs

     Maintenance:
- 1.5 – 3 g/d po ÷ BID – TID

*Infuse at ≤ 0.1 mmol/kg/hr
MAX: 0.2 mmol/kg/hr
*Infusion may cause hypotension

(con't)

Electrolyte Disturbances (con't)
Hyperphosphatemia: Serum $PO_4 > 4.0$
mg/dl

Short term: Circumoral paresthesias, paresthesias of the digits, sx of tetany

Long term: Precipitation of $CaPO_4$ in non-osseous sites

Causes: Renal insufficiency, widespread cell necrosis, DKA, hypoparathyroidism, pseudohypoparathyroidism

Tx: Dietary restriction, phosphate binders i.e. aluminum containing antacids

- -

HYPEROSMOLAR HYPERGLYCEMIC NONKETOTIC COMA

- Occurs in non-insulin dependent diabetics
- Characterized by severe hyperglycemia, hyperosmolality, dehydration and **absence of ketoacidosis**
- Serum glucose levels are usually > 800 mg/dl (> 1000 mg/dl are seen)
- Precipitating factors such as infection, MI, CVA, subdural hematoma, GI bleed, renal failure, newly diagnosed DM

S/S: Obtundation, N/V, extreme dehydration, neurologic defects – reversible hemiplegia or focal sz, tachycardia, polyuria

*Patient may be deficient 8 – 12 liters of fluid, 5 – 15 mEq/kg K^+, 50 – 100 mEq Ca^{++}, 50 – 100 mEq Mg^{++}, 70 –140 mmol PO_4

Tx:
- Fluid:
  - 0.9 NS for hypotension and to maintain UO @ 50 ml/hr
    *Usually 1 – 2 L over 1 – 2 hr
    *If patient has significant hypernatremia (155 mEq/L) or HTN, hypotonic saline (0.45 NS) should be used   (con't)

79

HHNC (con't)
- Δ to 0.45 NS once VS are stable
- Replace ½ the fluid deficit over the 1st 24 hr, the next ½ over the following 24 hr
  *Must replace the fluid slowly to avoid encephalopathy due to cerebral edema from fluid shifts

  To calculate fluid deficit:
  kg wt × 0.6 × % deficit = L of fluid
  *Use patient's normal weight
  *Use a deficit of 20 – 25%

- Hyperglycemia:
  - Vigorous IV hydration will decrease the serum glucose
  - Low dose insulin infusion at 1 – 2 U/hr to lower the glucose no > 75 – 100 mg/dl/hr
    *If glucose level is not lowering by 75 – 100 mg/dl/hr, ↑ insulin gtt up to 0.1 U/kg/hr
  - Add D_5W when glucose level is 250 – 300 mg/dl to avoid cerebral edema

*Too rapid correction of the hyperglycemia will cause cerebral edema (75% mortality rate), hypotension, acute tubular necrosis and vascular collapse

- Electrolytes
  - Na^+ will be replaced w/ the use of 0.9 NS and/or 0.45 NS
  - K^+: once adequate UO obtained, start replacing immediately or within 2 hr of initiating treatment, usually at a dose of 10 – 20 mEq/hr during the first 24 – 36 hr
  - Mg^{++}: monitor and replace PRN
  - HPO_4: monitor and replace PRN

*These patients are at risk for arterial and venous thrombosis, therefore use low-dose heparin or low molecular weight anticoagulants

- -

JONES CRITERIA FOR RHEUMATIC FEVER

1. Preexisting Group A Streptococcus infection

    Criteria:
    -   **F**ever > 101°F
    -   **A**ge 5 – 15 yo
    -   **N**ovember to May presentation
    -   **C**ervical adenopathy
    -   **U**RI absent
    -   **P**haryngitis
    *FAN CUP   (con't)

Jones Criteria for Rheumatic Fever (con't)
 # Criteria vs Risk of Group A Strep Infection:

1	0%
2 – 3	20%
4	40%
5	60%
6	75%

2. 2 or more major manifestations:
    -   carditis
    -   migratory polyarthritis
    -   CNS: Syndenham's chorea: involuntary, purposeless, rapid movements
    -   SQ nodules
    -   erythematous rash

OR

3. 1 major and 1 minor manifestation:
    -   temperature
    -   arthralgia
    -   ↑ acute phase reactants

- -

RANSON'S CRITERIA FOR ACUTE PANCREATITIS

At presentation:
1. Age > 55 yo
2. WBC > 16,000 µL
3. Glucose > 200 mg/dl
4. AST > 250 IU/L
5. LDH > 350 IU/L

Initial 48 hr:
1. Base deficit > 4 mEq/L
2. ↑ BUN > 5 mg/dl
3. Fluid Sequestration > 6 L
4. Ca^{++} < 8 mg/dl
5. Hct ↓ > 10%
6. PO_2 < 60 mmHg

0 – 2 criteria: < 5% mortality
3 – 4 criteria: ~ 15% mortality
5 – 6 criteria: ~ 40% mortality
7 – 8 criteria: ~ 100% mortality

- -

THYROTOXICOSIS/THYROID STORM

Causes: Grave's dz:
- Excess production of thyroid hormone
  *70 – 85% of cases

Toxic multinodular goiter:
- Seen in elderly with CHF, atrial fibrillation, tachydysrhythmias. Caused from the leakage of hormone from inflamed thyroid.

Exogenous causes:
- Ingestion 300 µg/d T_4 or > 100 µg/d T_3, amiodarone, K^+ iodide

S/S: Excessive diaphoresis, heat intolerance, weight loss despite ↑ appetite, diarrhea, tremor, dyspnea, tachycardia, hyperthermia (> 104°F = thyroid storm), staring or frightened look

Tx:
- Acetaminophen/cooling blanket
- IV fluids for hydration
- 25 – 50 mg chlorpromazine and 25 – 50 mg meperidine IV q 4 – 6 hr to achieve blockade of central thermoregulation centers
- IV digoxin for atrial fibrillation (higher doses PRN)
- Propylthiouracil: Load 600 – 1000 mg, then administer 200 – 500 mg q 4 hr PO/NG
- Propranolol 1 – 2 mg slow IV
  *MR 1 mg q 15 min
  *MAX: 10 mg
- Propranolol gtt for maintenance 5 – 10 mg/hr
  *Inhibits the peripheral transformation of T_4 to T_3
- Methimazole 20 mg q 4 hr
- Steroids if granulomatous dz, vitamin D toxicity or multiple myeloma

- -

TOTAL PARENTRAL NUTRITION

Requirements:

- Fluid: 30 – 35 ml/kg/d
- Calories: 30 – 35 kcal/kg/d
- Protein: 0.5 – 1.5 g/kg/d (up to 2 g/kg)
  *Use branched chain AA in liver failure
- Cal/N Ratio: 100 – 150 nonprotein Cal/g N or $\geq$ 25 Cal/g protein
- Electrolytes
  - Na^+ 2 – 4 mEq/100 ml H_2O metabolized
  - Cl^- 2 – 3 mEq/100 ml H_2O metabolized
  - K^+ 2 – 3 mEq/100 ml H_2O metabolized

*Electrolytes are usually added as a fixed amount w/ the other electrolytes
*If use > 20 mEq KPO_4 and > 20 mEq Ca^{++} gluconate, add L-cysteine to $\downarrow$ the pH of the solution to prevent precipitation of contents
*Acetate will cause alkalosis – good to use if patient has metabolic acidosis

Laboratory Studies:
- Glucose q 6 hr w/ coverage
  *Can add insulin to the TPN
- Daily: Electrolytes, Ca^{++}, Mg^{++}, HPO$_4^-$,
  CBC, BUN and Cr until stable,
  then q 3 d
- Daily: Weights and I & O's
- Weekly: LFT's, TG, PT/PTT, prealbumin,
  albumin

CALCULATIONS:
Amino Acids:
- 4.25% provides 0.17 kcal/ml

Dextrose:
- 10%   provides 0.34 kcal/ml
- 12.5% provides 0.43 kcal/ml
- 25%   provides 0.86 kcal/ml

Intravenous Fat Emulsion:
- 10% provides 1.1 kcal/ml
- 20% provides 2.0 kcal/ml

(con't)

TPN (con't)
FLUID CALCULATIONS:
Step 1:
Pt wt_____ kg × _____ml/kg/d = _____total volume

Step 2:
_____total volume – _____ml lipid/d = _____ml dextrose – AA solution volume/d

Step 3:
Total Volume ÷ 24 hr = _____ml/hr to infuse

CALORIE CALCULATIONS:
Dextrose sol'n: ___kcal/ml × ___ml = ___kcal
+
*From step 2 above

AA sol'n: ___kcal/ml × ___ml = ___kcal
+

IV Fat sol'n: ___kcal/ml × ___ml = ___kcal
=

TOTAL = _____ kcal//d

TOTAL ÷ kg wt = _____kcal/kg

- -

ABCIXIMAB (ReoPro)

Use: To prevent ischemic complications
during percutaneous coronary
intervention
*GPIIb/IIIa receptor antagonist

Dose: Adult: Load: 0.25 mg/kg IV bolus
10 – 60 min before
procedure

Infuse: 0.125 µg/kg/min for
12 – 24 hr
MAX: 10 µg/min

Contraindications:
- Active internal bleeding
- Recent (within 6 weeks) GI/GU bleed of
clinical significance
- CVA within 2 years or CVA w/ significant
neurological deficit
- Bleeding diathesis
- Administration of oral anticoagulants
within 7 d – unless PT ≤ 1.2 times the
control
- Thrombocytopenia < 100,000
- Recent (within 6 weeks) major surgery or
trauma
- Intracranial neoplasm, AVM or aneurysm
- Severe uncontrolled HTN
- Use of IV Dextran w/ intervention
- Use cautiously w/ ASA and heparin

- -

ACETYLCYSTEINE (Mucomyst)

Use: Tx of acetaminophen poisoning
Note: Liver toxicity can occur w/ 140
mg/kg of acetaminophen in
children and 7.5 g in adults.

10 – 15 g of acetaminophen can
produce hepatic failure, 25 g can
be fatal in adults.

Dose: Adult: PO: 140 mg/kg followed by 70
mg/kg q 4 hr × 17 doses

IV: 150 mg/kg in 200 ml D_5W
over 15 min. Then, infuse
50 mg/kg in 500 ml D_5W
over 4 hr. Then infuse 100
mg/kg in 1000 ml D_5W
over 16 hr. Total dose
over 20 hr is 300 mg/kg.
*IV use is NOT FDA
approved
*∅ use oral preparations
of acetylcysteine for IV,
unless the oral
preparation is pyrogen
free

Peds: Same dose w/ ↓ fluid

APAP: Therapeutic 10 – 30; Toxic > 70

Use: Mucolytic

Dose: Adult and Peds: 1 – 10 ml of 20% sol'n
or 2 – 20 ml of 10%
sol'n aerosolized q
2 – 6 hr PRN
*Can induce coughing
or bronchospasm

- - - - - - - - - - - - - - - - - - - -

ADENOSINE (Adenocard)

Use: PSVT, WPW not associated w/ atrial
fibrillation
*If WPW w/ atrial fibrillation, use
lidocaine (3 – 5 mg/kg) or procainamide
(15 mg/kg over 20 min) to slow the rate
*Cardiac filling is usually impaired at
rates above 180 beats per minute

Dose: Adult: 6 mg bolus over 2 seconds
followed by rapid NS flush.
Wait 1 – 2 min for conversion.
If PSVT persists, repeat w/ 12
mg bolus followed by rapid NS
flush.
*MR 12 mg × 2, if required

Peds: 0.1 mg/kg bolus followed by
rapid NS flush. Repeat w/
double dose if no response.
MAX: 12 mg/dose
(con't)

Medications – Adenosine (con't)
Contraindication: Asthma – will cause
bronchoconstriction

SE: Facial flushing, SOB, chest pressure, HA,
transient dysrhythmias including asystole.
PSVT recurrence after medication is as
high as 50 – 60%.

*Administer 50% of usual dose for patients
with a central line or for those patients on
on dipyridamole (dipyridamole ↑ the
half-life of adenosine)

*∅ use w/ cardiac transplant patients

*Not effective or higher doses may be needed
if patient is on xanthine derivatives i.e.
theophylline, caffeine

*Adenosine dilates coronary arteries
– –

ALBUMIN (Human) USP 5%, 25%
Use: 5% (expands plasma volume
0.5 – 1.5 × that of the albumin
amount infused)
Hypovolemic shock, hemodialysis
hypoalbuminemia, and
cardiopulmonary bypass

Use: 25% (expands plasma volume 4 – 5 ×
that of the albumin amount
infused)
Use is the same as for 5% and
also in patients w/ fluid overload,
ARDS, albumin loss from trauma,
acute nephrosis, acute liver failure
or ascites
*∅ use 25% albumin for
hypovolemic states since it pulls
the volume from the already
volume depleted interstitial fluid

Dose: Adult: 500 ml of 5% or 100 ml of 25%
PRN

Child: 12 – 20 ml of 5% sol'n/kg IV q
10 – 30 min PRN or 2.5 – 5 ml
of 25% sol'n/kg q 10 – 30 min
PRN

Infant: 1 g/kg of 5% or 25%

SE: Fever, chills, rash, N/V, tachycardia,
hypotension, hypertension, pulmonary
edema

NOTE: wnl serum colloid oncotic pressure
(COP) is 17 – 25 mmHg
*5% albumin has a COP of 20 mmHg
*25% albumin has a COP of 70 mmHg

- - - - - - - - - - - - - - - - - - - -

ALBUTEROL (Proventil)
β_2 agonist

Use: Bronchodilation, hyperkalemia

Nebulized Dose:
   Adult/Child > 12 yrs: 2.5 – 5.0 mg q 6 hr

   Child 5 – 12 yr: 2.5 mg q 4 – 6 hr PRN

   Child 1 – 5 yr: 1.25 – 2.5 mg q 4 – 6 hr

   Neonate/Infant < 1yr: 0.05 – 0.15 mg/kg
                          q 4 – 6 hr

   Continuous aerosol: 0.5 mg/kg/hr
                        MAX: 15 mg/hr

*Alternatively: Neonate to Child < 12 yr:
                 0.01 – 0.03 ml/kg (8 – 25
                 µg/kg) q 4 – 6 hr
- -

AMINOCAPROIC ACID (Amicar)

Use: Enhances hemostasis when fibrinolysis
contributes to bleeding.
Hyperfibrinolysis or hyperplasminemia.

Distinguish between 1° fibrinolysis and DIC:
- platelet ↓ in DIC, wnl in 1° fibrinolysis
- protamine paracoagulation test is (+) in
  DIC, (–) in 1° fibrinolysis
- euglobin clot lysis test is wnl in DIC,
  abnormal in 1° fibrinolysis

***MUST use heparin along w/ aminocaproic
acid if patient has DIC**

***Rapid injection will cause hypotension,
N/V/D, HA, dizziness**

*STOP administration if ↑ CPK

Dose: IV: 16 – 20 ml (4 – 5 g) in 250 ml NS
over 1 hr. Then 4 ml (1 g)/hr in 50
ml NS × 8 hr or until bleeding is
controlled
PO: 5 g during 1st hour then 1.25 g/hr
× 8 hr

Alternate dosing: 100 mg/kg over 1 hr then
10 – 20 mg/kg/hr

*Doses > 30 g/24 hr are NOT recommended

- -

AMINOPHYLLINE

Use: Bronchodilation

Dose: All ages: 6 mg/kg IV over 20 min
$\quad\quad\quad\quad$ *Each 1.2 mg/kg ↑ serum
$\quad\quad\quad\quad$ theophylline level by 2 mg/L

$\quad\quad$ Maintenance:
- $\quad$ > 12 yo: 0.7 mg/kg/hr IV
- $\quad$ 9 – 12 yo: 0.9 mg/kg/hr IV
- $\quad$ 1 – 9 yo: 1 – 1.2 mg/kg/hr IV
- $\quad$ 6 mo – 1 yr: 0.6 – 0.7 mg/kg/hr IV
- $\quad$ 6 wks – 6 mo: 0.5 mg/kg/hr IV
- $\quad$ Neonates: 0.2 mg/kg/hr IV

*Therapeutic levels
- $\quad$ Asthma: 10 – 20 mg/L
- $\quad$ Neonatal apnea: 6 – 13 mg/L

- - - - - - - - - - - - - - - - - - - -

AMIODARONE (Cordarone)

Use: Ventricular and supraventricular
$\quad\quad$ arrhythmias

Dose: Adult: Load: 150 mg IV over 10 min

$\quad\quad\quad\quad$ Infuse: 360 mg IV over 6 hr
$\quad\quad\quad\quad\quad\quad$ (1 mg/min)

Maintenance: 540 mg IV over
18 hr
(0.5 mg/min)
*After the first 24 hr, continue a
maintenance IV infusion of
720 mg/24 hr (0.5 mg/min)

*MAX: 1 – 2 g/d

Dose: Peds: Load: 5 mg/kg IV over 20 – 60
min
MAX: 15 mg/kg/d

SE: **Hypotension, pulmonary fibrosis,**
interstitial pneumonitis, ↑ liver enzymes,
↑ levels of other antiarrhythmics and
warfarin, blue-gray skin discoloration,
hyper-/hypothyroidism

Considerations:
- Administer via central line
- Metabolized in liver
- Monitor liver enzymes
- Prolonged half-life of 9 – 50 days
- -

AMRINONE LACTATE (Inocor)

Use: Phosphodiesterase inhibitor for the short term tx of systolic CHF unresponsive to digoxin, diuretics or vasodilators

Dose: Adult: Load: 0.75 mg/kg IV over 2 – 5 min
                       *MR × 1 in 30 min
        Infuse: 5 – 10 µg/kg/min

Peds: Same as adult except MR × 2

Neonate: Load: 0.75 mg/kg IV over 2 – 3 min
           Infuse: 3 – 5 µg/kg/min

*Total dose NOT to exceed 10 mg/kg/24 hr
*Concentration not to exceed 3 mg/ml
*∅ mix w/ dextrose
*NOT compatible w/ furosemide
*∅ administer to patients w/:
- aortic or pulmonary dz
- post MI
- caution w/ asthmatics
- patients taking disopyramide
- hypertrophic cardiomyopathy
*Synergistic w/ dobutamine
*Protect from light

SE: N/V, thrombocytopenia, abdominal pain, chest pain, arrhythmias, hypotension, hepatotoxicity

- -

ATENOLOL (Tenormin)

β_1 selective antagonist

Use: To reduce cardiovascular mortality and
risk of reinfarction in patients w/ acute MI

Adult Dose: 5 mg IV over 5 min. MR 5 mg IV
in 10 min. 50 mg PO 10 min
after last IV dose followed by 50
mg PO in 12 hr.

- -

ATRACURIUM (Tracrium)

Use: Nondepolarizing neuromuscular blocker

Dose: Adult/Child > 2 yo: 0.4 – 0.5 mg/kg IV
bolus
Maintenance: 0.08 – 0.10 mg/kg
q 12 – 45 min
Avg dose 12 – 35 mg

Children 1 mo to 2 yo: 0.3 – 0.4 mg/kg
Avg dose 1 – 5
mg
*Frequent maintenance doses PRN

Continuous Infusion (Adult/Child): 2 – 15
µg/kg/min
Average: 5 – 9
µg/kg/min

(con't)

99

Medications – Atracurium (con't)
SE: Prolonged apnea

*NOT compatible w/ alkaline sol'n i.e.
thiopental, barbiturates, NaHCO$_3$
*∅ mix w/ LR
*Eliminated in plasma

Duration: 20 – 35 min

Reversal: Neostigmine or edrophonium
co-administered w/ atropine

- - - - - - - - - - - - - - - - - - - -

ATROPINE
Use: Bronchospasm

Dose: Adult: 0.4 – 2.0 mg in 3 ml NS via
nebulizer

Child: 0.025 – 0.05 mg/kg in 2.5 ml NS
via nebulizer
MIN DOSE: 0.25 mg
MAX DOSE: 1 mg q 6 – 8 hr

- - - - - - - - - - - - - - - - - - - -

BETAMETHASONE (Celestone)

Use: Prevent neonatal RDS by administration
to the mother between 24 and 35 weeks
gestation. Also ↓ incidence of IVH.

Dose: 12.5 mg IM, repeat in 12 – 24 hr
 *Alternatively, use dexamethasone,
 same dose and times

- -

CALCIUM CHLORIDE 10%

Use: Hypocalcemia, Ca^{++} channel blocker
overdose, hypermagnesemia,
hyperkalemia

Dose: Adult: 2 – 4 mg/kg (0.02 – 0.04 ml/kg)
 IV q 10 min

OR

250 – 500 mg IV q 10 min

Infant/Child: 20 mg/kg (0.2 ml/kg) IV q
 10 min

*∅ exceed 100 mg/min w/ IV infusion
*Extravasation may lead to necrosis
*Hyaluronidase may be helpful
*Precipitates arrhythmias in digoxin toxicity

- -

CALCIUM GLUCONATE 10%

Use: Hypocalcemia, Ca^{++} channel blocker overdose, hypermagnesemia, hyperkalemia

Dose: Adult: 5 – 15 g/24 hr IV/PO ÷ q 6 hr

Child: 200 – 500 mg/kg/24 hr IV/PO ÷ q 6 hr

Infant: 200 – 500 mg/kg/24 hr IV ÷ q 6 hr
400 – 800 mg/kg/24 hr PO ÷ q 6 hr

Neonate: 200 – 800 mg/kg/24 hr IV ÷ q 6 hr

*∅ use w/ scalp veins
*Tx extravasation w/ hyaluronidase
*Precipitates arrhythmias in digoxin toxicity

- -

CEFTRIAXONE (Rocephin)

Use: Antibiotic, 3rd generation cephalosporin

Dose: Adult: 1 – 2 g/24 hr IV ÷ q 12 – 24 hr
MAX DOSE: 4 g/24 hr

Uncomplicated GC: 125 – 250 mg IM × 1 dose

Chancroid: 250 mg IM × 1

Meningitis: 100 mg/kg/24 hr IV ÷ q
12 – 24 hr
MAX DOSE: 4 g/24 hr

Dose: Infant/Child: 50 – 75 mg/kg/24 hr IV ÷
q 12 – 24 hr

Meningitis: 100 mg/kg/24 hr IV ÷ q
12 – 24 hr
MAX DOSE: 4 g/24 hr

Dose: Neonate: 25 – 50 mg/kg/24 hr IV ÷ q
12 – 24 hr

- -

CHLORAL HYDRATE (Noctec)
Use: Sedation
  Adult: 250 mg PO or PR TID
  Child: 8.3 mg/kg PO or PR TID
    MAX: 500 mg TID

Use: Insomnia
  Adult: 500 mg – 1000 mg PO or
    PR 15 – 30 min hs
  Child: 50 mg/kg PO or PR
    MAX: 1 g single dose

- -

CISATRACURIUM (Nimbex)
Use: Nondepolarizing neuromuscular blocker
*Eliminated in plasma

Dose: Adult: Load: 0.15 mg/kg IV
Infuse: 0.5 – 10 μg/kg/min

Child 2 – 12 yo: Load: 0.1 mg/kg IV
Infuse: 0.5 – 10
μg/kg/min

Duration: 45 – 120 min

*Monitor for malignant hyperthermia
*Higher doses may be required in burn
patients
- - - - - - - - - - - - - - - - - - - -

DANTROLENE (Dantrium)
Use: Malignant hyperthermia due to
anesthesia, succinylcholine, or
antipsychotic medications

Dose: Adult/Child: 1 – 2 mg/kg IV, repeat
PRN to MAX
accumulative dose
of 10 mg/kg, then
continue 4 – 8 mg/kg/24
hr PO ÷ q 6 hr × 3 days
- - - - - - - - - - - - - - - - - - - -

DEXAMETHASONE (Decadron)

Use: Cerebral edema

Dose: Adult: 10 mg (phosphate) IV; then
        4 – 6 mg IM q 6 hr × 2 – 4 days;
        taper after sx subside

Child: 1 – 2 mg/kg IV × 1
Maintenance: 1 – 1.5 mg/kg/24 hr
        ÷ q 4 – 6 hr

Use: Croup

Dose: Child: 0.6 mg/kg IM × 1

OR

0.25 – 0.5 mg/kg IM/IV q 6 hr
PRN

Use: Meningitis
    *Use is still controversial. Consult
    Infectious Disease.
    *Administer 15 – 20 min before 1st dose
    of antibiotic to ↓ neurologic
    complications in **bacterial meningitis**

Dose: Child > 6 weeks: 0.6 mg/kg/24 hr IV ÷
        q 6 hr × 4 days

(con't)

Medications – Dexamethasone (con't)
Use: Prevent neonatal RDS by administration
   to the mother between 24 and 35 weeks
   gestation. Also ↓ incidence of IVH.

Dose: 12.5 mg IM and repeat in 12 – 24 hr
   *Alternatively, use betamethasone,
   same dose and times
- -

DEXMEDETOMIDINE (Precedex)
α_2 agonist

Use: Sedation of initially intubated patients
   in the ICU setting

Dose: Adult: 1 µg/kg IV over 10 min

   Infuse: 0.2 – 0.7 µg/kg/hr

Mix: 2 ml of dexmedetomidine in 48 ml
   0.9% NS

SE: Bradycardia, sinus arrest, hypotension,
   HTN, nausea, atrial fibrillation

*∅ Use for > 24 hrs
- -

DIAZEPAM (Valium)

Use: Sedation, muscle relaxation

Dose: Adult: 2 – 10 mg IV/IM q 3 – 4 hr PRN

Child: 0.04 – 0.2 mg/kg IV/IM q
2 – 4 hr
MAX DOSE: 0.6 mg/kg within
an 8 hr period

Use: Seizures, status epilepticus

Dose: Adult: 5 – 10 mg IV q 10 – 15 min
MAX TOTAL DOSE: 30 mg

Child > 1 mo: 0.2 – 0.5 mg/kg IV q
15 – 30 min
MAX TOTAL DOSE:
< 5 yo: 5 mg
≥ 5 yo: 10 mg

Neonate: 0.3 – 0.75 mg/kg IV
q 15 – 30 min × 2 – 3 doses

*May stop the convulsion but it may not stop
the seizure. Phenytoin or phenobarbital may
be indicated.
*May be reversed w/ flumazenil

- -

DIAZOXIDE (Hyperstat)

Use: Rapid, emergency reduction of BP in cases of malignant hypertension

Dose: Adults/Children: 1 – 3 mg/kg IV bolus (up to MAX of 150 mg) q 5 – 15 min until adequate response is seen
*MR @ 4 – 24 hr intervals PRN

*Rapid IV push within 30 sec for maximum effect
*FOR IV USE ONLY

SE: Sz, paralysis, arrhythmias, MI, shock

- -

DIGOXIN (Lanoxin)

Use: To slow ventricular response in rapid atrial fibrillation, atrial flutter and for CHF

Dose: Adult: Load: 0.5 – 1.0 mg/d IV/IM/PO ÷ q 12 hr
Maint: 0.125 – 0.5 mg IV/PO qd

> 2 yo: Load: 0.015 – 0.035 mg/kg/d
                  IV or 0.02 – 0.04
                  mg/kg/d PO ÷ q 8 hr
     Maint: 0.012 mg/kg/d PO ÷
                  q 12 hr

1 mo to 2 yo: Load: 0.03 – 0.05
                  mg/kg/d IV or
                  0.035 – 0.06
                  mg/kg/d PO ÷
                  q 8 hr
     Maint: 0.01 – 0.02
                  mg/kg/d PO ÷ q
                  12 hr

Neonate: Load: 0.02 – 0.03 mg/kg/d
                  IV or 0.025 – 0.035
                  mg/kg/d PO ÷ q 8 hr

     Maint: 0.01 mg/kg/d PO ÷ q
                  12 hr

Premie: Load: 0.015 – 0.025 mg/kg/d
                  IV ÷ q 8 hr

     Maint: 0.01 mg/kg/d ÷ q
                  12 hr

*Consideration: Low K^+ ↑ toxicity
*Monitor levels in patients w/ renal or hepatic impairment

- - - - - - - - - - - - - - - - - - - -

109

DIGOXIN IMMUNE FAB (Digibind)

Use: Digoxin overdose

S/S: Bradycardia, $2°$ AVB, $3°$ AVB, VT, VF,
Hyperkalemia – $\varnothing$ give Ca^{++}

Dose: [(serum dig concentration $\times$ kg wt) $\div$
100] $\times$ 40 = mg dose
Infuse over 30 min w/ 0.22 micron filter
or IV bolus if cardiac arrest imminent
or $K^+ > 5.0$

*Monitor serum K^+ levels since digibind
causes hypokalemia*

*1-vial (40 mg) binds approximately 0.6 mg
digoxin*

Dilute: 4 ml SWI/vial = 10 mg/ml
35 ml SWI/vial = 1 mg/ml

# of digoxin tabs ingested*	Digibind mg	Dose # vials
25	340	8.5
50	680	17
75	1000	25
100	1360	34
150	2000	50
200	2680	67

*0.25 mg tablets or 0.2 mg Lanoxicaps

Child: First, determine total body digoxin load
(TBL) in mg:

TBL (mg) = [serum digoxin level
(ng/ml) × 5.6 × kg wt] ÷ 1000, OR
TBL (mg) = mg digoxin ingested × 0.8

Then, calculate dose of digoxin
immune Fab (mg): Fab (mg) =
TBL × 66.7 to be infused IV over
15 – 30 min through 0.22 micron filter

- -

DILTIAZEM (Cardizem)

Use: Atrial-fibrillation/flutter NOT associated
w/ WPW or short P-R syndrome; PSVT;
AV nodal reentrant tachycardia; WPW;
short P-R syndrome

Dose: Adult: 0.25 mg/kg bolus over 2 min
(20 mg avg dose)
- If response is inadequate, wait 15 min
and rebolus @
- 0.35 mg/kg (25 mg avg dose)
- Infuse 5 – 15 mg/hr

Dilute: 125 mg (25 ml) in 100 ml
5 mg/hr = 5 ml/hr

(con't)

Medications – Diltiazem (con't)

```
* 5 mg/hr = 180 mg/day PO
  7 mg/hr = 240 mg/day PO
 11 mg/hr = 360 mg/day PO
```

Contraindications: Sick Sinus Syndrome,
                    2° or 3° AVB w/o pacer,
                    hypotension, cardiogenic
                    shock, recent IV doses of
                    β-blockers

*↑ digoxin levels
*∅ use for > 24 hr
*Controls the rate in 90% of patients
*Produces less myocardial depression than
  verapamil in patients w/ LV dysfunction

- -

DIPHENHYDRAMINE (Benadryl)
Use: Antihistamine, allergic reaction

Dose: Adult: 10 – 50 mg/dose q 6 – 8 hr
              IV/IM/PO
              MAX DOSE: 400 mg/2 hr

      Child: 5 mg/kg/24 hr ÷ q 6 hr IV/IM/PO
              MAX DOSE: 300 mg/24 hr

*For anaphylaxis or phenothiazine overdose:
  1 – 2 mg/kg IV slowly

- -

DOBUTAMINE (Dobutrex)
β_1 agonist, mild β_2

Use: R and/or L systolic heart failure, chronic
CHF, right ventricular wall MI, during
cardiac surgery

*Rapid acting inotropic agent. ↑ CO, SV, renal
blood flow. SVR ↑ w/mild ↑ in BP.

Dose: Adult/Child: 2.5 – 20 µg/kg/min
MAX DOSE: 40 µg/kg/min

Contraindications: Hypertrophic
cardiomyopathy

*NOT indicated for diastolic dysfunction
*Half-life 2 min
*Ø mix w/ alkaline solutions
*Synergistic w/ amrinone or milrinone

- -

DOLASETRON (Anzemet)
Use: Post-operative nausea

Dose: Adult: 12.5 mg IV q 6 hr PRN

Child: 0.35 mg/kg IV q 6 hr PRN

(con't)

Medications – Dolasetron (con't)
Use: Prevent pruritis after narcotic
administration

Dose: Adult: 12.5 mg IV q 6 hr PRN
- - - - - - - - - - - - - - - - - - - -

DOPAMINE (Intropin)
dopaminergic, β, α agonist

Use: Tx of hypotension $2°$ sepsis, neurogenic
shock, cardiogenic shock, augment
cardiac output in patients w/ renal
insufficiency

Dose: Adult/Child:
- Low (dopaminergic): 0.5 – 2.0 µg/kg/min
  - ↑ myocardial contractility, CO and
    renal perfusion w/o ↑ HR or SVR;
    ↑ urinary Na^+ and H_2O excretion

- Moderate (β_1, β_2): 2 – 10 µg/kg/min
  - ↑ CO, SVR, pulmonary vascular
    resistance and BP

- High (α_1, α_2): 10 – 50 µg/kg/min
  - Causes potent vasoconstriction w/
    diminished renal and mesenteric
    perfusion

Contraindications: Uncontrolled
                   tachyarrhythmias, VF,
                   uncorrected hypovolemia,
                   pheochromocytoma,
                   tachycardic patients

1° Action: direct β-agonist
2° Action: release norepinephrine from
           synaptic nerve terminals leading
           to ↑ BP

*MUST wean slowly since dopamine depletes
the norepinephrine stores and may lead to
hypotension
*NOT indicated for patients w/ diastolic
dysfunction
*∅ mix w/ alkaline sol'n

tyrosine → dopa → dopamine →
norepinephrine
- -

DPT KIDS COCKTAIL
Use: Sedation

Demerol 1 – 2 mg/kg
Phenergan 0.5 – 1.0 mg/kg
Thorazine 0.5 – 1.0 mg/kg

Administer as single IM injection
- -

115

DROPERIDOL (Inapsine)

Use: N/V, sedation, premedication for
anesthesia

Dose: Adult: 0.625 – 2.5 mg IV PRN q
4 – 6 hr
Premed: 2.5 – 10 mg IV

Child: 0.03 – 0.07 mg/kg IV over 2
min. If needed, may give
0.1 – 0.15 mg/kg
MAX INITIAL DOSE: 2.5 mg

*Administer PRN q 4 – 6 hr for N/V

- - - - - - - - - - - - - - - - - - - -

EDROPHONIUM (Tensilon)

Use: Termination of PAT or PSVT associated
w/ WPW unresponsive to digitalis
glycosides

Dose: Adult: IV bolus 5 – 10 mg

Use: Reversal of NMB-nondepolarizing,
myasthenia gravis (DOC =
pyridostigmine). AChE blocker.

Dose: Adult: 10 mg IV bolus over 30 – 45 sec
MR q 5 – 10 min
MAX DOSE: 40 mg

Child > 34 kg: 2 mg IV bolus. If no
response within 45 sec,
give 1 mg q 45 sec
MAX DOSE: 10 mg

Child < 34 kg: 1 mg IV bolus. If no
response within 45 sec,
give 1 mg q 45 sec
MAX DOSE: 5 mg

*Have atropine on hand
*Ø **administer for reversal of
succinylcholine**

- -

ENALAPRILAT (Vasotec)
Use: Antihypertensive, ACE inhibitor

Dose: Adult (not on diuretic): 1.25 mg IV over
5 min q 6 hr

Adult (on diuretic): 0.625 mg IV over 5
min. Repeat in 1 hr
if needed, then 1.25
mg IV over 5 min q
6 hr

Child: 0.005 – 0.01 mg/kg IV q
8 – 24 hr

- -

EPHEDRINE (Efedron)

α_1, α_2, β_1, β_2 agonist

Use: Hypotension – less SE for fetus than dopamine

Dose: Adult: 5 – 25 mg IV @ 10 mg/min
q 3 – 4 hr
MAX: 150 mg/24 hr

Child: 3 mg/kg/d IV ÷ q 4 – 6 hr
MAX: 3 mg/kg/d

Mix: Add 9 ml for total of 10 ml. Administer 2.5 – 5.0 mg IV (0.5 – 1.0 ml)

SE: Potent stimulation of CNS
*Hypoxia, hypercapnia, acidosis may ↓ effectiveness or ↑ adverse reactions. Correct before administering ephedrine.

Antidote for ephedrine:
- Hypotension: IV fluids
  Vasopressors contraindicated
- Hypertension: phentolamine 2 – 5 mg IV/IM
- Sz: diazepam
- Cardiac arrhythmias: β-blockers
  *Watch for exacerbation of HTN, since the α-receptors will be uninhibited

- - - - - - - - - - - - - - - - - - - -

118

EPINEPHRINE (Adrenaline)

α_1, α_2, β_1, β_2 agonist

Use: Hypotension and/or bradycardia
*Effectiveness is ↓ w/ acidosis
*β-effect: 0.05 – 0.5 µg/kg/min

Dose: Adult/Child: 0.1 – 1.5 µg/kg/min by
continuous infusion
titrated to response
Neonate: 0.05 – 1.0 µg/kg/min

Use: As a drip in an arrest situation

Dose: 30 mg of 1:1000 epinephrine mixed in
250 ml D_5 or NS run at 100 ml/hr will
infuse 1 mg q 5 min

Use: Anaphylactic shock

Mix: 1 mg in 500 ml for a concentration of
2 µg/ml infused at 60 ml/hr
MAX RATE: 240 ml/hr

Use: Epistaxis

Mix: 0.25 ml of 1:1000 epinephrine mixed w/
20 ml 4% lidocaine placed in pledget

- -

EPTIFIBATIDE (Integrilin)

Use: Acute coronary syndromes
  *GPIIb/IIIa receptor antagonist
  *Use w/ heparin and ASA

Dose: Adult: Load 180 µg/kg over 2 min
      MAX: 22.6 mg, then infuse
        2 µg/kg/min × 72 hrs
      MAX: 15 mg/hr

Use: Adjunct to percutaneous coronary
  intervention

Dose: Adult: Load 135 µg/kg IV bolus just
      prior to procedure, then infuse
      0.5 µg/kg/min × 20 – 24 hrs
      after intervention

Contraindications:
- Active internal bleeding
- Hemorrhagic CVA or CVA within 30 days
- Bleeding diathesis
- Concomitant use of other parentral GPIIb/IIIa receptor antagonists
- Thrombocytopenia < 100,000
- Recent (within 6 weeks) major surgery or trauma
- Intracranial neoplasm, AVM or aneurysm
- Severe uncontrolled HTN
- Dialysis or creatinine ≥ 2

- - - - - - - - - - - - - - - - - - -

ESMOLOL (Brevibloc)

$\beta_1 > \beta_2$ agonist

Use: Short term tx of PSVT, acute aortic
dissection to keep MAP 60 – 80 mmHg
*Half-life 9 min

Dose: Adult: 500 µg/kg loading dose over
1 min initially, followed by
50 µg/kg/min infusion for 4 min

If no response within 5 min, give 2nd
loading dose of 500 µg/kg over 1 min
and ↑ infusion to 100 µg/kg/min for 4
min

If no response, repeat loading dose of
500 µg/kg over 1 min and ↑ infusion
rate by 50 µg/kg/min increments
(not to exceed 200 ug/kg/min)

As therapeutic endpoint is achieved,
eliminate loading doses and ↓ dosage
increments to 25 µg/kg/min

Dilution: Add 5 g to 500 ml D_5W, NS or
LR after removing 20 ml from the
500 ml
Final concentration: 10 mg/ml or
10,000 µg/ml

(con't)

Medications – Esmolol (con't)
Dose: Peds: 100 – 500 µg/kg over 1 min

   Maintenance infusion: 25 – 100
                           µg/kg/min

   If inadequate response, may
   readminister loading dose above, and/or
   ↑ maintenance dose by 25 – 50
   µg/kg/min q 5 – 10 min

   Usual maintenance dose range:
   5 – 500 µg/kg/min

SE: Hypotension, nausea, bronchospasm,
    CHF, N/V

*Morphine may ↑ esmolol level by 46%

Contraindications: Uncompensated CHF,
                    pulmonary edema,
                    cardiogenic shock,
                    bradycardia, 2° or 3° AVB

Toxicity/OD: Bradycardia, severe vertigo or
              syncope, severe drowsiness,
              dyspnea, cyanotic nail beds or
              palms, sz
              *NOTIFY PHYSICIAN

*∅ use for > 48 hr and wean slowly
- -

ETOMIDATE (Amidate)

Use: Induction of general anesthesia

Dose: Adult/Child > 10 yo: 0.2 – 0.6 mg/kg
IV over 30 – 60
sec

*Trismus occurs in 20% of patients – if this
occurs, use more etomidate
*Muscle movement can be ↓ w/ 100 μg
fentanyl in the adult or 1 μg/kg in children

SE: Myoclonus, tonic movements, transient
apnea, eye movement, N/V, cortisol
suppression, ↓ ICP, ↓ IOP

Duration: 3 – 5 min

*Etomidate is a hypnotic agent and ∅ have
any analgesic properties
- -

FENTANYL (Sublimaze)

Use: Narcotic analgesic, sedation

Dose: Adult: Low dose: 2 µg/kg IV over 3 – 5 min

Mod dose: 2 – 20 µg/kg IV over 3 – 5 min, then 25 – 100 µg IV PRN

High dose: 20 – 50 µg/kg IV over 3 – 5 min then 25 µg to ½ initial loading dose IV PRN

Peds: 1 – 3 µg/kg/dose IV over 3 – 5 min or IM q 30 – 60 min PRN

Continuous infusion (adult and peds):
Start @ 1 µg/kg/hr and titrate to response to a maximum of 3 µg/kg/hr

*Rapid injection or high doses may cause respiratory depression and chest wall muscle rigidity, reversible w/ neuromuscular blocker

*May be reversed w/ naloxone
- Mix 0.4 mg w/ 9 ml NS (40 µg/ml). Administer 40 µg IV over 2 min while assessing patient response. MR × 2.

- -

FLUMAZENIL (Romazicon)

Use: Benzodiazepine sedation reversal

Dose: Adult: 0.2 mg IV over 15 sec.
If desired LOC not obtained
within 45 sec, give 0.2 mg IV
q 60 sec
MAX DOSE: 1 mg in 20 min or
3 mg in 60 min

*Repeat tx may be given no > q 20 min
*MAX amount to be given in 5 min: 1 mg

Peds:
- Initial dose 0.01 mg/kg
MAX: 0.2 mg
- Then, 0.005 – 0.01 mg/kg
(MAX: 0.2 mg) given q 1 min
to a maximum total cumulative
dose of 1 mg
*Doses may be repeated in 20
min up to a maximum of 3 mg
in 1 hr

SE: Sz, N/V, vertigo

*The administered benzodiazepine may last
longer than the flumazenil dose

- -

FOSPHENYTOIN (Cerebyx)
*All dosing is expressed as phenytoin sodium equivalents (PE)

Use: Status epilepticus

Dose: 5 yo – Adult: 15 – 20 mg PE/kg IV

Maintenance: 4 – 6 mg PE/kg/d IV/IM

Use: Prevention or treatment of sz

Dose: 5 yo – Adult: 10 – 20 mg PE/kg IV
Maintenance: 4 – 6 mg PE/kg/d IV/IM

*∅ administer at a rate > 150 mg PE/min

- -

FUROSEMIDE (Lasix)
Use: Peripheral edema, pulmonary edema, some HTN states

Dose: Adult: 20 – 120 mg slow IV
MR up to 1000 mg total

Peds: 0.5 – 2.0 mg/kg q 6 – 12 hr
MAX: 6 mg/kg/dose

Neonate: 0.5 – 1.0 mg/kg q 8 – 24 hr
          MAX : 2 mg/kg IV, 6 mg/kg PO

Continuous infusion (adults and peds):
0.05 – 0.75 mg/kg/hr titrated to response
*Use when > 80 mg is needed to produce
 desired diuresis

- - - - - - - - - - - - - - - - - - - -

GLUCAGON
Use: Antihypoglycemic agent

Dose: Adult: 0.5 – 1.0 mg IV/IM/SQ q 20 min
        PRN
        *May also be used for
        esophageal spasms

Child: 0.03 – 0.1 mg/kg IV/IM/SQ q
        20 min PRN
        MAX DOSE: 1 mg/dose

Infant/Neonate: 0.025 – 0.3 mg/kg q
        30 min PRN
        MAX: 1 mg/dose

- - - - - - - - - - - - - - - - - - - -

HEPARIN
Use: Anticoagulation

Dose: Adult: 80 U/kg IV bolus followed by
continuous infusion of
18 U/kg/hr

Check PTT 6 hr after start of infusion and
titrate as follows:

PTT (sec)	Bolus Dose	Infusion
< 35	80 U/kg	↑ by 4 U/kg/hr
35 – 45	40 U/kg	↑ by 2 U/kg/hr
46 – 70	------------------	------------------
71 – 90		↓ by 2 U/kg/hr
> 90	------------------	Stop for 1 hr, then ↓ by 3 U/kg/hr

Child: 50 U/kg IV bolus followed by
10 – 25 U/kg/hr infusion OR
50 – 100 U/kg IV q 4 hr

Use: Anticoagulation in patient w/ MI and
thrombolytics

Dose: Adult: 60 U/kg IV bolus (MAX: 4000U)
followed by 12 U/kg/hr
(MAX: 1000 U/hr)

*GOAL: PTT 50 – 70 for 48 hrs

128

*Monitor for
- heparin induced thrombocytopenia
- ↑ K^+ due to heparin induced aldosterone suppression (usually seen within a few days after initiating therapy)
- ↑ serum alanine aminotransferase (ALT) levels (usually seen within 5 – 10 d after initiating therapy)

*ACT (Activated Clotting Time) is measured if using high doses of heparin i.e. cardiovascular surgery or ECMO
*WNL: 150 – 200 sec

Use: Cardioembolic CVA
   *∅ anticoagulate until CT scan @ 48 hr
   - If CT @ 48 hr shows:
      - Hemorrhagic transformation: delay anticoagulants
      - No hemorrhage but large CVA or patient is hypertensive: delay anticoagulants
      - No hemorrhage but small to moderate size CVA and wnl BP: anticoagulate according to your institution's policy

*May be reversed w/ protamine sulfate

- - - - - - - - - - - - - - - - - - - -

HYDRALAZINE (Apresoline)

Use: Hypertensive emergency

Dose: Adult: 20 – 40 mg slowly by IV
q 3 – 6 hr PRN
*Switch to PO antihypertensives
ASAP

Peds: 0.1 – 0.2 mg/kg slow IV q
2 – 6 hr PRN
*Not to exceed 20 mg/dose

SE: Reflex tachycardia, pleural effusion,
headache, palpitations, angina, N/V/D

- -

HYDROCORTISONE (Solu-Cortef)
Use: Status asthmaticus

Dose: Adult: 100 – 500 mg IV q 6 hr

Child: Load: 4 – 8 mg/kg IV
MAX: 250 mg

Maintenance: 8 mg/kg/d IV ÷ q
6 hr

Use: Shock

Dose: Adult: 50 mg/kg IV repeated in 4 hr
Repeat 50 mg/kg q 24 hr PRN

Child: 0.16 – 1.0 mg/kg IV qd – BID

- -

HYDROMORPHONE (Dilaudid)
Use: Narcotic analgesic

Dose: Adult: 1 – 4 mg IV q 4 – 6 hr PRN

Peds: 0.015 mg/kg IV q 3 – 4 hr

Continuous Infusion: 0.0075 mg/kg/hr
titrated as
necessary for
pain relief

Use: Patient controlled analgesia

Basal Rate: 0.0015 – 0.003
mg/kg/hr
Intermittent Bolus: 0.0015 – 0.0045
mg/kg bolus w/
lockout interval
of 6 – 15 min

(con't)

131

Medications – Hydromorphone (con't)
*May be reversed w/ naloxone
- Mix 0.4 mg w/ 9 ml NS (40 µg/ml), administer 40 µg IV over 2 min while assessing patient response. MR × 2.

- - - - - - - - - - - - - - - - - - - -

IBUTILIDE (Corvert)
Use: Rapid conversion of atrial fibrillation or atrial flutter of recent (< 90 days) onset

Dose: Adult > 60 kg: 1 mg IV infused over
                                         10 min
          Adult: < 60 kg: 0.01 mg/kg (0.1 ml/kg)
                                         IV infused over 10 min

*If the arrhythmia is not converted within 10 min after the end of the first infusion, a second infusion of equal strength can be administered over 10 min
*Mix in D_5W or NS

SE: Arrhythmias, hypotension, bundle branch block, CHF, syncope

*MUST monitor ECG for @ least 4 hr due to risk of Torsades de Pointes (2%)
*Patients w/ atrial fibrillation > 2 – 3 d duration should be adequately anticoagulated for @ least 2 weeks before conversion attempted

- - - - - - - - - - - - - - - - - - - -

INDOMETHACIN (Indocin)
Use: Closure of a hemodynamically
significant PDA

Dose: Neonate < 48 hr: 0.2 mg/kg IV over
20 – 30 min followed
by two doses of
0.1 mg/kg @
12 – 24 hr intervals

Neonate 2 – 7 days: 0.2 mg/kg IV over
20 – 30 min
followed by two
doses of
0.2 mg/kg @
12 – 24 hr
intervals

Neonate > 7 d: 0.2 mg/kg IV over
20 – 30 min followed by
two doses of 0.25
mg/kg @ 12 – 24 hr
intervals

SE: Sz, CHF, GI bleeding, acute renal failure,
hemolytic anemia, aplastic anemia,
agranulocytosis, thrombocytopenic
purpura, Stevens-Johnson syndrome,
anaphylaxis, angioedema
- -

IPRATROPIUM BROMIDE (Atrovent)

Use: Bronchospasm

Dose: Adult: 500 µg q 6 – 8 hr aerosolized

Child: < 2 yo: 250 µg/dose q 6 – 8 hr aerosolized

Child: ≥ 2 yo: 250 – 500 µg/dose q 6 – 8 hr aerosolized

- - - - - - - - - - - - - - - - - - - -

ISOPROTERENOL (Isuprel)

β_1, β_2 agonist

Use: Heart block, ventricular arrhythmias, shock

Dose: Adult: 2 – 5 µg/min
*MAX: 10 µg/min

Dose: Peds: 0.1 – 2.0 µg/kg/min
*Start 0.1 µg/kg/min and titrate by 0.1 µg/kg/min q 5 – 10 min until desired effect or toxicity occurs
*MAX: 2 µg/kg/min

134

SE: Flushing, ventricular arrhythmias,
    profound hypotension, cardiac arrest,
    tachycardia, myocardial ischemia,
    palpitations, Adams-Stokes sz

*Ventricular arrhythmias more likely if
 HR > 130
*∅ use for asystole
*∅ use for cardiac arrest unless the arrest
 is due to bradycardia from heart block
- -

KETAMINE (Ketalar)
Use: General anesthetic, sedation

*Causes dissociative anesthesia: sedation,
amnesia, immobility
*Patient appears awake but is unconscious
and will not feel pain

Dose: Adult: 1.0 – 4.5 mg/kg IV over 60 sec
                or 3 – 8 mg/kg IM
                *Usually 1 – 2 mg/kg lasts
                10 – 15 min

        Continuous Infusion: 0.1 – 0.5 mg/min

(con't)

135

Medications – Ketamine (con't)

Peds: 0.25 – 1.0 mg/kg IV over 60 sec
or 2 – 5 mg/kg IM

Continuous Infusion: 5 – 20 µg/kg/min

*To maintain sedation, repeat @ ½ of full initial dose
*Rate of infusion should **not** exceed 0.5 mg/kg/min or be administered in less than 60 sec

SE: Bronchodilation, tonic/clonic movements, respiratory depression, hallucinations, ↑ BP, ↑ HR due to ↑ catecholamines, ↑ cerebral blood flow leading to ↑ ICP

*Maintain quiet, dim environment as the patient comes out of the anesthesia to decrease risk of hallucinations

Contraindicated: Elevated ICP, HTN, aneurysms, thyrotoxicosis, CHF, angina, psychotic disorders

- - - - - - - - - - - - - - - - - - - -

LABETALOL (Normodyne)

α, β antagonist

Use: Severe HTN associated w/ adequate CO
*Useful in aortic dissection and intracranial hemorrhage management
*$\downarrow$ SVR and BP w/o $\uparrow$ HR or CO
*$\varnothing$ $\uparrow$ ICP

Dose: Adult: 20 mg over 2 min
MR 40 – 80 mg q 10 min
MAX DOSE: 300 mg/dose

Infusion: 2 mg/min, $\uparrow$ to titrate to response up to 100 mg/hr
MAX: 2400 mg/d

Child: 0.3 – 1.0 mg/kg IV q 10 min PRN
MAX DOSE: 20 mg/dose

Infusion: 0.4 – 1.0 mg/kg/hr
MAX of 3 mg/kg/hr

SE: Hypotension, myocardial depression, bronchospasm

- -

LEVALBUTEROL (Xopenex)

Pure β_2 agonist

Use: Bronchodilation for patients that are unable to tolerate the side effects of albuterol

Dose: Adult/Child/Infant: ¼ albuterol dose

*2.5 mg albuterol = 0.63 mg levalbuterol
5.0 mg albuterol = 1.25 mg levalbuterol
7.5 mg albuterol = 1.88 mg levalbuterol
10 mg albuterol = 2.50 mg levalbuterol

- -

LORAZEPAM (Ativan)

Use: Seizures

Dose: Adult: 2 – 4 mg slow IV over 2 – 5 min
MR in 5 – 15 min
MAX DOSE: 8 mg in 12 hr

Child/Infant/Neonate: 0.05 – 0.1 mg/kg
slow IV over
2 – 5 min
MR 0.05 mg/kg ×
1 in 10 – 15 min

138

Use: Sedation

Dose: Adult: 1 – 4 mg IV q 4 – 6 hr PRN

       Continuous Infusion: 0.1 mg/kg/hr
                          *Usual dose is
                          1 – 5 mg/hr

       Child: 0.05 mg/kg IV/PO q 4 – 8 hr

*May be reversed w/ flumazenil

- - - - - - - - - - - - - - - - - - - -

MAGNESIUM
Use: Hypomagnesemia

Dose: Adult/Child: 25 – 50 mg/kg q 4 – 6 hr
                    × 3 – 4 doses

Use: AMI

Dose: Adult: 2 g over 30 – 60 min

Use: Rate control in atrial fibrillation

Dose: Adult: 2 g over 5 – 15 min, then infuse
            6 g over 6 hr

(con't)

Medications – Magnesium (con't)
Use: Tocolytic

Dose: 4 – 6 g bolus over 15 – 20 min,
        followed by 2 g/hr

Mix: 40 g in 1000 ml LR or NS for a
      concentration of 0.04 g/ml

Administer: 100 – 150 ml (4 – 6 g) over
             15 – 20 min, followed by 50 ml/hr
             *Total dose not to exceed
              30 – 40 g daily

*Monitor respirations, deep tendon reflexes
 and BP

*STOP infusion if:
-        **Respiratory rate**
         < 12 breaths per min
-        **Patellar reflex is absent**
-        **< 100 ml UO over 4 hr**

Goal: Maintain Mg^{++} level between
          4 – 8 mEq/L

*If Cr > 1.3 administer the full loading dose
and ↓ the maintenance infusion dose by ½

Levels and Associated Toxicity
10 mg/dl – loss of DTR's
15 mg/dl – respiratory depression
> 25 mg/dl – cardiac arrest

Overdose Tx: Ca^{++} gluconate 1 g over @
least 3 min or CaCl 10%
2 – 4 mg/kg

- - - - - - - - - - - - - - - - - - - -

MANNITOL (Osmitrol)
Use: Reduction of ↑ ICP

Dose: Adult/Child > 12 yo: 1.5 – 2.0 g/kg as a
15 – 25% IV sol'n
over 30 – 60 min

Child < 12 yo: 0.25 g/kg/dose IV over
20 – 30 min. May ↑
gradually to 1 g/kg/dose
if needed. May
administer furosemide
1 mg/kg concurrently or
5 min before mannitol.

*Reduction in ICP occurs in 15 min and lasts
3 – 6 hr

Use: Test dose for marked oliguria or
suspected inadequate renal function

Dose: Adult/Child > 12 yo: 200 mg/kg as a
25% IV sol'n over
3 – 5 min

(con't)

Medications – Mannitol (con't)
NOTE: Diuresis is adequate if 30 – 50 ml
urine/hr is excreted over 2 – 3 hr; if
diuresis is inadequate, a second test
dose is given. If still no diuresis after
the second test dose, mannitol should
not be continued.

Dose: Child < 12 yo: 0.2 g/kg/dose IV
MAX 12.5 g over
3 – 5 min

NOTE: If there is no diuresis within 2 hr,
discontinue mannitol

- -

MEPERIDINE (Demerol)
Use: Narcotic, analgesic

Dose: Adult: 50 – 150 mg IV q 3 – 4 hr PRN
Infusion: 15 – 35 mg/hr

Child: 1.0 – 1.5 mg/kg q 3 – 4 hr PRN
MAX DOSE: 100 mg

Contraindication: Cardiac arrhythmias,
asthma, ↑ ICP

*∅ use if patient taking MAO inhibitor, i.e.
phenelzine, tranylcypromine, isocarboxazid
*May be reversed w/ naloxone
- -

METARAMINOL (Aramine)

α_1, α_2, β_1 agonist

Use: Severe hypotension in the critically ill
      patient

1° Action: Synthetic catecholamine that
           causes general vascular
           constriction, ↑ BP and cardiac
           stimulation
2° Action: R release of norepinephrine

Dose: Adult: 0.5 – 5.0 mg IV as a single IV
              injection
      Infusion: Start @ 5 µg/kg/min and
                titrate to maintain desired BP
                Mix: 100 mg in 250 ml D_5W

      Peds: 0.01 mg/kg as a single IV
            injection
      Infusion: 2 mg/50 ml D_5W adjusting
                rate to maintain BP

SE: Hypovolemia due to vasodilation and
    capillary leak syndrome, arrhythmias,
    cardiac arrest

*To tx extravasation: Infiltrate site promptly w/
10 – 15 ml NS containing 5 – 10 mg
phentolamine. Use a fine gauge needle.

- - - - - - - - - - - - - - - - - - -

143

METHYLENE BLUE

Use: Tx methemoglobinemia, amyl nitrate
     inhalation or nitrate overdose

S/S: Cyanosis, chocolate brown blood

MetHgb Levels
> 3% – abnormal
> 40% – tissue ischemia
> 70% – lethal

Tx: Adult/Child:
- 100% O_2/NRB
- Methylene blue 1% sol'n
   1 – 2 mg/kg over 5 min

*MR @ 1 hr intervals up to 7 mg/kg
*Improvements seen within 30 – 60 min
*∅ exceed 7 mg/kg since methylene blue may
  cause methemoglobinemia

- -

METHYLPREDNISOLONE
(Solu-Medrol)
Use: Status asthmaticus

Dose: Adult: 40 – 250 mg IV q 4 – 6 hr

      Child: Load: 2 mg/kg IV
             Maintenance: 2 mg/kg/d IV ÷ q
                     6 hr

Use: CNS trauma within the first 4 hr of injury

Dose: Adult/Child: 30 mg/kg bolus over 15 min followed in 45 min by a continuous infusion of 5.4 mg/kg/hr × 23 hr MAX RATE: 500 mg/min

- - - - - - - - - - - - - - - - - - - -

METOPROLOL (Lopressor)
β_1 selective antagonist

Use: Early intervention in acute MI

Dose: Adult: 5 mg IV over 1 min. MR @ 2 min intervals × 2 additional doses for total of 15 mg. 50 mg PO 15 min after last IV dose.

- - - - - - - - - - - - - - - - - - - -

MIDAZOLAM (Versed)
Use: Conscious sedation

Dose: Adult < 60 yo: 1.0 – 2.5 mg slow IV over 2 min. Wait 2 min. If adequate sedation is not achieved, give 0.5 – 1.0 mg slow IV q 4 min up to 5 mg total dose.   (con't)

Medications – Midazolam (con't)

    Adult > 60 yo: 1.0 – 1.5 mg slow IV
                    over 2 min. Wait 2 min.
                    If adequate sedation is
                    not achieved, give
                    0.5 – 1.0 mg slow IV q
                    4 min up to 3.5 mg total
                    dose.

    Child: 0.05 – 0.1 mg/kg over 2 min
           MR 0.05 mg/kg q 2 – 3 min
           PRN
           MAX TOTAL DOSE: 0.2 mg/kg

Midazolam Continuous Infusion:
Adult: Load: 0.025 – 0.1 mg/kg IV

    Maintenance:
        Light sedation: 0.03 – 0.04
                mg/kg/hr
        Deep sedation: 0.06 – 0.15
                mg/kg/hr

Infant/Child: 0.5 – 3.0 µg/kg/min titrated to
              effect

Neonates: 0.2 – 1.0 µg/kg/min titrated to
          effect

Use: Intubation or sedation after intubation, induction for general anesthesia

Dose: Adult < 55 yo: 0.3 – 0.35 mg/kg IV
                          over 20 – 30 sec

       Adult > 55 yo: 0.15 – 0.25 mg/kg IV
                          over 20 – 30 sec

*May be reversed w/ flumazenil
*Avoid using in patient receiving erythromycin or ↓ dose by 50 – 75%

- -

MILRINONE (Primacor)
Use: Phosphodiesterase inhibitor for the short term tx of systolic CHF unresponsive to digoxin, diuretics or vasodilators. Action is to ↑ CO, relaxes vascular smooth muscle, ↓ preload and afterload.
    *20 times more potent than amrinone w/ less side effects

Dose: Adult: Load 50 µg/kg slowly over 10 min followed by a continuous IV infusion of 0.375 – 0.75 µg/kg/min

Dose: Peds: Load 50 – 75 µg/kg followed by a continuous infusion of 0.5 – 0.75 µg/kg/min   (con't)

147

Medications – Milrinone (con't)
SE: Ventricular arrhythmias

*Usual daily dose is 0.77 mg/kg
*Use cautiously in patients w/ atrial fibrillation
  or atrial flutter since the drug decreases AV
  conduction time
*Typically drug is given w/ digoxin and
  diuretics
*Incompatible w/ furosemide
*Synergistic w/ dobutamine
- -

MIVACURIUM (Mivacron)
Use: Nondepolarizing neuromuscular blocker
      *Eliminated in plasma

Dose: Adult: Load: 0.15 mg/kg IV
               Infuse: 4 – 10 µg/kg/min

      Child 2 – 12 yo: Load: 0.2 mg/kg IV
                       Infuse: 5 – 31
                                µg/kg/min

Duration: 15 min

*Ø administer to patients w/ low plasma
  psuedocholinesterase
*Causes histamine release
*Reversed w/ neostigmine
- -

MORPHINE

Use: Narcotic, analgesic

Dose: Adult: 2 – 15 mg IV q 2 – 6 hr PRN
   Infusion: Load 15 mg IV, then
      0.8 – 10 mg/hr

   Child/Infant: 0.1 – 0.2 mg/kg q
      2 – 4 hr PRN
   Infusion: 0.025 – 2.6 mg/kg/hr

Use: Neonatal analgesia or tetralogy spells

   Dose: 0.05 – 0.2 mg/kg slow IV q 4 hr
   Infusion: 0.01 – 0.02 mg/kg/hr

Use: Patient controlled analgesia
   Basal Rate: 0.01 – 0.02 mg/kg/hr
   Intermittent bolus: 0.0015 – 0.0045
         mg/kg w/ a
         lockout interval of
         6 – 15 min

*May be reversed w/ naloxone
- Mix 0.4 mg w/ 9 ml NS (40 µg/ml),
  administer 40 µg IV over 2 min while
  assessing patient response. MR × 2.
- - - - - - - - - - - - - - - - - - - -

NALOXONE (Narcan)

Use: Narcotic antagonist

Dose: Adult: 0.4 – 2.0 mg IV q 2 – 3 min up
to 10 mg

Child > 20 kg or > 5 yr: 2 mg/dose q
2 – 3 min PRN

Child < 20 kg/Neonate: 0.1 mg/kg q
2 – 3 min PRN

Continuous Infusion (all ages): 0.005 mg/kg
loading dose followed by
an infusion of
0.0025 – 0.16 mg/kg/hr

Use: ↓ pruritis due to narcotics

Dose: 1 – 2 µg/kg/hr (will not affect analgesia)

Use: ↓ sedation if patient on PCA pump

Dose: Mix 0.4 mg w/ 9 ml NS (40 µg/ml).
Administer 40 µg IV over 2 min while
assessing patient response. MR × 2.

- -

NEOSTIGMINE (Prostigmin)
Use: Reversal of NMB-nondepolarizing
agents

Dose: Adult: 0.5 – 2.5 mg IV slowly
(0.5 mg/min)
MAX DOSE: 5 mg/dose
*Pretreat w/ 0.6 – 1.2 mg
atropine IV

Child: 0.025 – 0.08 mg/kg slowly
*Pretreat w/ 0.011 mg/kg
atropine IV

Infant: 0.025 – 0.1 mg/kg slowly
*Pretreat w/ 0.011 mg/kg
atropine IV

***∅ administer for the reversal of
succinylcholine. Neostigmine will
prolong the action of succinylcholine.**

*See physostigmine if you need a drug to
cross the blood brain barrier if tx TCA,
atropine or anthistamine overdose

*Reversed w/ atropine
- -

NICARDIPINE (Cardene)

Use: HTN

Mix: 25 mg in 240 ml NS or D_5W
(concentration: 0.1 mg/ml)

Dose: Adult: 0.5 – 15 mg/hr

Titrate: Gradual ↓ BP: Start @ 50 ml/hr
(5 mg/hr) and ↑ by 25
ml/hr (2.5 mg/hr) q 15
min
MAX: 150 ml/hr
(15 mg/hr)

Rapid ↓ BP: Same dosing as above
except titrate q 5 min
MAX: 150 ml/hr
(15 mg/hr)

*After desired BP reached, ↓ gtt gradually to
30 ml/hr (3 mg/hr)
*Metabolized by liver, ↑ coronary perfusion,
↑ CO
*∅ **use w/ diagnosis of advanced aortic
stenosis**

*20 mg PO q 8 hr = 0.5 mg/hr
30 mg PO q 8 hr = 1.2 mg/hr
40 mg PO q 8 hr = 2.2 mg/hr
- - - - - - - - - - - - - - - - - - - -

NITROGLYCERIN (NTG, Tridil)

Use: Vasodilator, antihypertensive, acute MI, angina

Dose: Adult: 5 – 200 µg/min
  *Begin @ 5 µg/min and ↑
  by 5 µg/min q 3 – 5 min
  *If no improvement @
  20 µg/min, ↑ dose by
  10 – 20 µg/min q 3 – 5 min until
  pain relief, hypotension, or
  200 µg/min reached

Adult: Bolus for CP: 12.5 – 25 µg PRN

  Bolus for HTN: 100 – 800 µg
  PRN

Child: 0.25 – 0.5 µg/kg/min
  *↑ by 0.5 – 1.0 µg/kg/min q
  3 – 5 min PRN
  MAX DOSE: 5 µg/kg/min

Contraindicated: ↑ ICP, glaucoma, severe anemia

*May cause ethanol or propylene glycol toxicity. If suspected measure serum osmolarity.

- -

NITROPRUSSIDE
(Nipride, SNP)
Use: Antihypertensive, vasodilator, $\downarrow$ SVR

Dose: Adult/Child: 0.2 – 0.5 µg/kg/min titrated
to effect
MAX DOSE:
10 µg/kg/min

*Usual dose is 0.5 – 2.0 µg/kg/min in CHF and
2 – 5 µg/kg/min in HTN

SE: $\uparrow$ ICP, thiocyanate toxicity,
methemoglobinemia, cyanide toxicity

*Add sodium thiosulfate 10 mg for q 1 mg SNP
to prevent cyanide toxicity
*Protect from light
*Monitor thiocyanate levels if used for > 48 hr
*Thiocyanate levels should be < 50 mg/L
*Cyanide levels $\leq$ 0.1 – 0.2 µg/ml

S/S Cyanide Toxicity
CNS: Disorientation, agitation, lethargy, sz,
coma, cerebral death
Cardiovascular: Initial $\uparrow$ HR and BP followed
by $\downarrow$ BP, shock and lethal
cardiac arrhythmias
Respiratory: Early tachypnea followed by
apnea
- - - - - - - - - - - - - - - - - - - -

NOREPINEPHRINE (Levophed)

α_1, α_2, β_1 agonist

Use: Hypotension and during cardiac arrest
    *Produces venous and arterial
    vasoconstriction, ↑ BP, CO, PAP and
    coronary blood flow
    *High doses lead to ↓ CO and may
    cause renal failure

Dose: Adult: 8 – 12 µg/min initially, then
            2 – 4 µg/min maintenance
            titrated to BP response
           *Dilute 4 mg in 250 ml D_5W or
            D_5NS
            Concentration: 16 µg/ml
            2 µg/min = 7.5 ml/hr
           *MAX: 80 ug/min

      Peds: 0.05 – 1.0 µg/kg/min titrated to
           effect
          MAX: 2 µg/kg/min

Contraindications: Thrombosis, pregnancy,
                   hypoxia, hypercarbia,
                   hypotension 2°
                   hypovolemia

*Incompatible w/ blood or plasma
*D/C infusion gradually to prevent hypotension
*Protect from light

(con't)

Medications – Norepinephrine (con't)
*To tx extravasation, infiltrate site promptly w/
10 – 15 ml NS containing 5 – 10 mg
phentolamine. Use a fine gauge needle.
*10 ml phentolamine may be added to each
liter of sol'n to help prevent phlebitis or
necrosis if the drug extravasates. Pressor
effect is not affected

- -

OCTREOTIDE (Sandostatin)
Use: Variceal bleeding

Dose: Adult: Bolus: 25 – 50 µg IV
            Infuse: 25 – 50 µg/hr

SE: Nausea, diarrhea, abdominal pain or
    discomfort, loose stools, HA, pain or
    burning at site of injection

- -

ONDANSETRON (Zofran)
Use: Antiemetic, prevent post-operative N/V

Dose: Adult: 4 mg IV over 2 – 5 min q
            6 hr PRN

    Child > 3 yo: 0.15 mg/kg IV over
                2 – 5 min
                MAX: 4 mg

- -

OXYTOCIN (Pitocin)

Use: Labor stimulation and induction
      GOAL: Contractions q 3 min and
              Montevideo units between
              210 – 250
    *If Montevideo units > 280, d/c oxytocin
    to prevent uterine rupture
    *Must have @ least a 30 min tracing w/
    fetal reactivity before starting the gtt

Dose: 1 – 2 mU/min
      ↑ by 1 – 2 mU q 15 – 30 min until
      wnl contraction pattern established,
      then ↓ dose
      MAX: 24 mU/min

Mix: 30 units in 500 ml NS or D_5W
      (concentration 60 mU/ml)
      *1 ml/hr = 1 mU/min

*If contractions occur < 2 min apart and are
> 50 – 65 mmHg on the monitor, if they last
60 – 90 sec or longer, or significant change in
FHR, stop infusion, turn the patient to L side
and notify the physician

*Montevideo Unit: Sum of the mmHg
peaks of each contraction in a 10 min
period

(con't)

Medications – Oxytocin (con't)
Use: Reduction of post-partum hemorrhage
     after expulsion of placenta

Dose: 10 – 40 units infused @ rate necessary
     to control hemorrhage
       *Usual dose 20 – 40 mU/min
       MAX: 40 mU/min

Mix: 10 – 40 units in 1000 ml NS or D_5W

Use: Incomplete or inevitable abortion

Dose: 10 – 20 mU/min

Mix: 10 units in 500 ml NS or D_5W

*$MgSO_4$ PRN to relax the myometrium

- -

PANCURONIUM (Pavulon)
Use: Nondepolarizing neuromuscular blocker

Dose: 1 mo – Adult: 0.04 – 0.1 mg/kg IV

       Maintenance: 0.015 – 0.1 mg/kg IV q
               30 – 60 min

Neonate: 0.02 mg/kg IV

Maintenance: 0.05 – 0.1 mg/kg q
0.5 – 4 hr PRN

Duration: 60 min

Contraindications: Tachycardia, dehydration

*Antidote: neostigmine w/ atropine

- - - - - - - - - - - - - - - - - - -

PENTOBARBITAL (Nembutal)
Use: Barbiturate coma

Dose: Adult/Child: Load: 10 – 15 mg/kg IV
over 1 – 2 hr

Maintenance: 1 – 3
mg/kg/hr

*Therapeutic serum level: 20 – 40 mg/L

- - - - - - - - - - - - - - - - - - -

PHENOBARBITAL (Luminal)
Use: Seizures, status epilepticus

Dose: Adult: 10 – 20 mg/kg IV slowly
MAX TOTAL: 600 mg

Maintentance: 60 mg IV q 3 hr (con't)

Medications – Phenobarbital (con't)

Child/Infant/Neonate: 15 – 20 mg in
single or ÷ dose.
May give
additional
5 mg/kg q
15 – 30 min
MAX TOTAL:
30 mg/kg

Maintenance:
- > 12 yo: 1 – 3 mg/kg/d ÷
q 12 – 24 hr
- 6 – 12 yo: 4 – 6 mg/kg/d ÷
q 12 – 24 hr
- 1 – 5 yo: 6 – 8 mg/kg/d ÷
q 12 – 24 hr
- Neonates: 3 – 5 mg/kg/d ÷
q 12 – 24 hr

*Give slow IVP, no faster than 1 mg/kg/min
*Therapeutic levels: 15 – 40 mg/L

Use: Hyperbilirubinemia

Dose: Child < 12 yo: 3 – 12 mg/kg/d ÷ q
8 – 12 hr

Use: Sedation

Dose: Child: 6 mg/kg/d ÷ qd – BID

- - - - - - - - - - - - - - - - - - - -

PHENTOLAMINE (Regitine)

α_1, α_2 antagonist

Use: Extravasation antidote for dopamine, ephedrine, epinephrine, norepinephrine, phenylephrine

Dose: Adult/Child/Infant: Make a sol'n of 0.5 – 1.0 mg/ml w/ NS. Inject 1 – 5 ml (in 5 divided doses) SQ around site of extravasation. MAX TOTAL DOSE: 0.1 – 0.2 mg/kg or 5 mg total

Dose: Neonate: Make a sol'n of 0.25 – 0.5 mg/ml w/ NS. Inject 1 ml (in 5 divided doses) SQ around site of extravasation. MAX TOTAL DOSE: 0.1 mg/kg or 2.5 mg total

*Use a 27 – 30 gauge needle w/ multiple small injections
*To prevent phlebitis or necrosis due to extravasation, 10 mg phentolamine can be added to each liter of norepinephrine. Pressor effect is not affected.

- - - - - - - - - - - - - - - - - - - -

PHENYLEPHRINE
(Neo-Synephrine)
α_1 agonist

Use: Maintenance of BP in shock and drug
      induced hypotension

Dose: Adult: Bolus: 0.1 – 0.5 mg IV q
                         10 – 15 min PRN
           Infusion: Start @ 100 – 180
                       µg/min. After BP
                       stabilized, ↓ to
                       40 – 60 µg/min
         Alternatively: Start @ 1 – 4
                       µg/kg/min and
                       titrate to effect

          IM/SQ: 2 – 5 mg q 1 – 2 hr
                PRN

      Peds: Bolus: 5 – 20 µg/kg IV q 10 – 15
                   min PRN
           Infusion: 0.1 – 0.5 µg/kg/min
                  titrated to effect

          IM/SQ: 0.1 mg/kg q 1 – 2 hr PRN

SE: HA, reflexive bradycardia, tremors, CP,
     sweating, short runs of VT, paresthesias

*Antidote is phentolamine

- - - - - - - - - - - - - - - - - - - -

PHENYTOIN (Dilantin)

Use: Seizures, status epilepticus

Dose: Adult: 10 – 15 mg/kg IV
              MAX TOTAL: 1.5 g
              *∅ exceed 50 mg/min

        Maintenance: 100 mg IV/PO q
                        6 – 8 hr

(desired – measured) × kg wt × 0.8 = mg dose
to give if patient levels are low

        Child: 15 – 20 mg/kg IV
              *∅ exceed 1 mg/kg/min in infants
              *∅ exceed 50 mg/min in children

        Neonate: Start w/ 5 mg/kg/d IV/PO ÷ q
                12 hr
                *Usual range is
                  5 – 8 mg/kg/d ÷ q 8 – 12 hr
                *∅ exceed 0.5 mg/kg/min in
                neonates

*For IV extravasation use lidocaine,
 nitroglycerin paste or regitine
*NOT compatible w/ D_5W, use 0.9% NS
- -

PHYSOSTIGMINE(Antilirium)

Use: Reverses CNS effects due to overdose
of drugs (belladonna, phenothiazines,
TCA, antihistamines, atropine) causing
anticholinergic syndrome

Action: AChE blocker causing ↑ muscle tone,
bronchial/ureteral constriction,
bradycardia,↑ salivation, lacrimation,
sweating, CNS stimulation
*Crosses blood brain barrier

S/S: "Mad as a hatter, red as a beet, blind as
a bat, hot as a hare, dry as a bone": oral
dryness and burning, speech and
swallowing difficulties, ↓ GI motility,
thirst, blurred vision, photophobias,
mydriasis, skin flushing, tachycardia,
fever, urinary urgency, delirium,
hallucinations, cardiovascular collapse.

Dose: Adult: 0.5 – 2.0 mg IV slowly @
1 mg/min
*MR q 20 min until response,
then 1 – 4 mg IV q 30 – 60 min
PRN as symptoms recur

Child: 0.02 mg/kg IV slowly q
5 – 10 min
MAX DOSE: 2 mg

SE: Restlessness, N/V/D, abdominal
    cramping, bradycardia, bronchospasm,
    sz

*If overdose, give atropine 0.5 mg for q mg of
physostigmine just given

- -

POTASSIUM
Use: Hypokalemia

Tx: Adult: 10 – 15 mEq KCl/hr IV

Sliding Scale:
3.6 – 3.9 20 mEq IV/PO
3.5 – 3.2 40 mEq IV/PO
3.1 – 2.8 50 mEq IV/PO
< 2.8   Call Physician

    Child: 1 – 2 mEq KCl/kg IV slowly @
            0.5 – 1.0 mEq/kg/hr
            MAX: 20 mEq/hr

*10 mEq raises serum K^+ by 0.1 mmol/L
*If K^+ < 2.0 administer 30 – 40 mEq KCl/hr
 monitoring ECG and potassium level closely

- -

PRALIDOXIME (Protopam)

Use: Antidote for organophosphate poisoning

Dose: Adult: $1 - 2$ g $\times 1$ IV/IM/SQ
MR in $1 - 2$ hr if muscle
weakness is not relieved

Peds: $20 - 40$ mg/kg $\times 1$ IV/IM/SQ
MR in $1 - 2$ hr if muscle
weakness is not relieved

*For IV administration, dilute to 50 mg/ml or
less and infuse over $15 - 30$ min
*May cause muscle rigidity, laryngospasm,
tachycardia after rapid IV infusion
*If pulmonary edema, give IVP over 5 min
MR in 1 hr
*Give atropine if cyanosis present
MR q $5 - 6$ min

***CONTRAINDICATED IN POISONING W/
SEVIN® (Commercially available
insecticide)***

PROCAINAMIDE (Pronestyl)
Use: PSVT, VT, VF

Dose: Adult: Bolus: 17 mg/kg @ 30 mg/min
until:
- arrhythmia suppressed
- QRS widens by 50% of
  baseline
- hypotension develops
- 17 mg/kg has been given

Infusion: 1 – 4 mg/min

*If renal patient ↓ loading dose to 12 mg/kg
and then use ½ of the maintenance dose

Peds: Bolus: 15 mg/kg over 30 – 60 min

Infusion: 20 – 80 μg/kg/min
MAX: 2 g/24 hr

*Therapeutic levels: 4 – 10 mg/L of
procainamide or 10 – 30 mg/L of
procainamide + NAPA levels combined

- -

PROPOFOL (Diprivan)

Use: Sedation – rapid acting

Dose: Adult: Load: 0.25 – 1 mg/kg
Maintenance:
- Light sedation:
  1 – 3 mg/kg/hr
  (17 – 50 µg/kg/min)
- Deep sedation:
  3 – 6 mg/kg/hr
  (50 – 100µg/kg/min)

Alternatively: Start infusion @ 5 µg/kg/min
and ↑ by 5 – 10 µg/kg/min q
5 min PRN until desired
sedation is achieved
*Use loading dose if needed

*Use ½ adult dose if patient > 55 yo

Use: Anesthesia or short-term procedural
sedation

Dose: Peds ≥ 3 yo: 1 – 3 mg/kg IV bolus

Infusion: 0.125 – 0.3 mg/kg/min

SE: Hypotension, ↓ ICP, HA, dizziness, tonic-
clonic movements, bradycardia, N/V,
HTN, apnea, fever

*Usually ↓ BP by 20 – 30%
*Produces sedation in 1 min and lasts
 4 – 8 min
*In obese patients use IBW
*∅ depress myocardium
*Not recommended in OB patients, breast
 feeding mothers, patient w/ ↑ ICP or impaired
 cerebral circulation
*Assess neurological and respiratory status qd
**NOT AN ANALGESIC – MUST PROVIDE
 PAIN CONTROL**

- -

PROPRANOLOL (Inderal)

β_1, β_2 non-selective antagonist

Use: Supraventricular and ventricular
      arrhythmias, tachyarrhythmias due to
      excessive catecholamine, HTN

Dose: Adult: 0.5 – 1.0 mg given q 5 min
               up to total of 5 mg

       Neonate/Child: 0.01 – 0.1 mg/kg IV
                       push over 10 min
                       MR q 6 – 8 hr PRN
                       MAX DOSE CHILD:
                       3 mg/dose
                       MAX DOSE
                       NEONATES:
                       1 mg/dose

- -

PROSTAGLANDIN E$_1$
(Alprostadil, Prostin VR)

Use: Vasodilator, maintain PDA – for palliation only of Tetralogy of Fallot, interrupted aortic arch, transposition of the great vessels, aortic coarctation, tricuspid atresia

Dose: Neonates: 0.05 – 0.1 µg/kg/min
↑ to 0.2 µg/kg/min if necessary
MAX DOSE: 0.4 µg/kg/min

Maintenance: When ↑ PaO$_2$ noted, ↓ immediately to lowest effective dose. Can be as low as 0.025 µg/kg/min but usually 0.01 – 0.05 µg/kg/min

SE: Sz, bradycardia, hypotension, tachycardia, cardiac arrest, DIC, apnea, flushing, fever, hypokalemia, apnea, ↓ platelet aggregation

*Usually effects are seen in 30 min in cyanotic lesions, several hours in acyanotic lesions

- -

170

PROTAMINE SULFATE

Use: Heparin antidote

Dose: 1 mg protamine will neutralize 115 U
porcine intestinal or 90 U beef lung
heparin

Consider time of heparin and antidote
administration:
- < 30 min: 1 – 1.5 mg/100 U IV
heparin
- 30 – 60 min: 0.5 – 0.75 mg/ 100 U
IV heparin
- ≥ 2 hr: 0.25 – 0.375 mg/100 U IV
heparin

MAX DOSE: 50 mg IV
MAX RATE: 5 mg/min diluted down to 1%
(10 mg/ml)

If on heparin and need reversal due to
bleeding:
1. Stop the heparin infusion
2. Administer 25 – 50 mg of protamine
3. Administer 10 U cryoprecipitate and/or
4. Administer 10 U FFP and/or
5. Administer 10 U platelets and/or
6. Administer 5 g IV or 0.1 mg/kg IV
aminocaproic acid loading dose over
30 – 60 min, then infuse 0.5 – 1.0 g/hr
× 8 hr or until bleeding is controlled

(con't)

Medications – Protamine (con't)
*Above may also be used for bleeding after thrombolytic therapy

*May cause hypotension, bradycardia, dyspnea and anaphylaxis. Monitor APTT.

*Hypersensitivity reaction is ↑ in patients w/ known hypersensitivity to fish, vasectomized or infertile males, or patients taking protamine-insulin products

– –

RANITIDINE (Zantac)
Use: H₂ antagonist to ↓ acid secretion

Dose: Adult: 50 mg IV q 6 – 8 hr
MAX DOSE: 400 mg/24 hr

Infant/Child: 2 – 4 mg/kg/24 hr ÷ q
6 – 8 hr
MAX DOSE: 6 mg/kg/24
hr

Neonate: 2 mg/kg/24 hr ÷ q 6 – 8 hr

*For a continuous infusion for all ages, administer daily IV dosage over 24 hr

Use: Stress ulcer prophylaxis

Dose: Adult: Load: 0.5 mg/kg IV over 30 min
Infuse: 0.125 mg/kg/hr

*↑ by 0.06 mg/kg/hr until gastric acid pH > 4.0

- -

RACEMIC EPINEPHRINE 2.25%
(Vaponephrine)
Use: Croup/Laryngotracheobronchitis

Dose:
< 20 kg:	0.25 ml
20 – 40 kg:	0.50 ml
> 40 kg:	0.75 ml

*0.05 – 0.1 ml/kg diluted in 2 – 3 ml NS
aerosolized over 15 min q 1 – 6 hr
USUAL MAX SINGLE DOSE: 0.5 ml

- -

RETEPLASE (Retevase)
Use: Thrombolytic for acute MI

Dose: Adult: Bolus #1: 10 U IV over 2 min
Wait 30 min, if no adverse
reactions, then
Bolus #2: 10 U IV over 2 min

Contraindications:
- Active internal bleeding or known bleeding diathesis
- History of CVA

- Intracranial or intraspinal surgery or trauma within 2 months
- Intracranial neoplasm, AVM, aneurysm
- Known bleeding diathesis
- Severe uncontrolled HTN

*Administer through separate line from other medications
Incompatible w/ heparin

- -

RITODRINE (Yutopar)

β_2 agonist

Use: Tocolytic

IV: Mix 150 mg in 500 ml of fluid
   (concentration 0.3 mg/ml)

Initial dose is 0.05 mg/min (10 ml/hr),
gradually ↑ by 0.05 mg/min q 10 min until
desired result is obtained or until maternal HR
↑ to 130 beats per min
*Usual effective dose is 0.15 – 0.35 mg/min

SE: HA, pulmonary edema, tachycardia, N/V,
    agranulocytosis, anaphylactic shock,
    hyperglycemia

Contraindications: < 20 weeks gestation;
                     antepartum hemorrhage;
                     eclampsia; severe pre-
                     eclampsia; intrauterine fetal
                     death; chorioamnionitis;
                     maternal cardiac dz, un-
                     controlled DM, pulmonary
                     HTN or hyperthyroidism

*D/C if HR > 140, FHR > 180, BP < 90/60, CP,
VPB's, PSVT, a-fibrillation, pulmonary edema
*Antidote: propranolol 0.5 – 1.0 mg slow IV or
           verapamil 5 – 10 mg slow IV

- - - - - - - - - - - - - - - - - - - -

ROCURONIUM (Zemuron)

Use: Nondepolarizing neuromuscular blocker

Dose: Adult/Ped: 0.6 – 1.2 mg/kg IV bolus

Maintenance bolus: 0.1 – 0.2 mg/kg IV
q 20 – 30 min

Maintenance Infusion: Start at 10 – 12
μg/kg/min and
titrate to
effect. Usual
range is 4 – 16
μg/kg/min in
adults.

SE: HTN, hypotension, tachycardia,
bronchospasm, N/V

**Duration: 30 – 40 min in children
20 – 94 min in adults**

*Reversed w/ neostigmine or edrophonium
- -

STREPTOKINASE (Streptase)

Use: Thrombolytic

Dose: Adult (AMI):
- 1.5 million IU over 60 min by IV infusion

Dose: Adult (Pulmonary Embolism):
- Load 250,000 IU over 30 min by IV infusion
- Then, 100,000 IU/hr for 24 – 72 hr by continuous IV infusion

Dose: Adult (Venous Thrombosis):
- Load 250,000 IU over 30 min by IV infusion
- Then, 100,000 IU/hr for 72 hr by continuous IV infusion

Dose: Adult (Arterial Thrombus or Embolism):
- Load 250,000 IU over 30 min by IV infusion
- Then, 100,000 IU/hr for 24 – 72 hr by continuous IV infusion

(con't)

Medications – Streptokinase (con't)
Contraindications:
- Active internal bleeding or known bleeding diathesis
- History of CVA
- Intracranial or intraspinal surgery or trauma within 2 months
- Intracranial neoplasm, AVM, aneurysm
- Known bleeding diathesis
- Severe uncontrolled HTN

SE: Hypotension, bleeding, bronchospasm, pulmonary edema, anaphylaxis, angioedema

*Reversed by aminocaproic acid
*To check for hypersensitivity: Give 100 IU intradermally. Wheal and flare within 20 min indicates that the patient is probably allergic.

-- -- -- -- -- -- -- -- -- -- -- -- -- --

SUCCINYLCHOLINE (Anectine)
Use: Depolarizing neuromuscular blocker

Dose: Adult: 0.3 – 1.5 mg/kg × 1
           MAX DOSE: 150 mg/dose

      Maintenance: 0.04 – 0.7 mg/kg
              IV q 5 – 10 min PRN

Infant/Child: 1 – 2 mg/kg IV × 1
MAX DOSE: 150
mg/dose

Maintenance: 0.3 – 0.6 mg/kg IV
q 5 – 10 min PRN
*Continuous infusion
NOT recommended

Duration: 5 – 10 min

Contraindications/Precautions:
- Severe burns or crush injuries and in patients w/ preexisting hyperkalemia or low plasma psuedocholinesterase
- Ø use if:
  - K^+ > 5.5 mEq/L
  - Burn victim within 3 d to 6 months of injury
  - Trauma victim w/ severe crush injuries within 3 d to 1 year of injury
  - Patient who has
    - Guillain-Barré
    - Amyotrophic Lateral Sclerosis (Lou Gehrig's dz)
    - Parkinson's dz
    - Spinal cord injury

(con't)

Medications – Succinylcholine (con't)

*May cause hyperkalemia in certain patients

*Serum K^+ ↑ 0.5 mEq/L on average
 (0.5 – 1.5 mEq/L)

*∅ cause hyperkalemia in patients w/ renal
 failure

*May cause **MALIGNANT HYPERTHERMIA**
 S/S:

- ↑ $EtCO_2$ – Most sensitive sign
- Tachycardia – Earliest sign
- Tachypnea
- Rigidity
- Cyanosis
- Hyperpyrexia – ONLY in 30% of the patients

TX:
- Dantrolene 2.5 mg/kg IV, repeat PRN to MAX cumulative dose of 10 mg/kg, then continue 4 – 8 mg/kg/24 hr PO divided q 6 hr × 3 days
- Rapid cooling, i.e. Iced saline, ice packs, iced lavage via gastric, peritoneal

*∅ use reversing agents since they
potentiate the effects of succinylcholine

- - - - - - - - - - - - - - - - - - - -

TENECTEPLASE (TNKase)
Use: Thrombolytic

Dose: Adult: Administer IV over 5 seconds

Kg Wt	TNKase (mg)
< 60	30
≥ 60 – < 70	35
≥ 70 – < 80	40
≥ 80 – < 90	45
≥ 90	50

Contraindications:
- Active internal bleeding or known bleeding diathesis
- History of CVA
- Intracranial or intraspinal surgery or trauma within 2 months
- Intracranial neoplasm, AVM, aneurysm
- Known bleeding diathesis
- Severe uncontrolled HTN

*NOT compatible w/ dextrose containing solutions
*Total dose NOT to exceed 50mg
*Tenecteplase converts fibrin bound plasminogen to plasmin
*Antidote is aminocaproic acid – use only if uncontrolled hemorrhage

- -

TERBUTALINE (Brethine)

β_2 antagonist

Use: Asthma

Dose: Adult/Child ≥ 12 yo: 0.25 mg SQ q
15 – 30 min PRN
× 2
MAX: 0.5 mg in a
4 hr period

Child ≤ 12 yo: 0.005 – 0.01 mg/kg SQ
q 15 – 20 min × 3
MAX: 0.4 mg/dose

Continuous Infusion: 2 – 10 µg/kg loading
dose followed by
0.1 – 0.4 µg/kg/min
MAX: 8 µg/kg/min

Use: Tocolytic

Dose: SQ: 0.25 mg SQ q 15 min, MR × 3 – 4

IV: Mix 5 mg in 500 ml LR or NS
(concentration: 10 µg/ml)
30 ml/hr = 5 µg/min
MAX DOSE: 80 µg/min

Contraindications: DM, HTN, cardiac dz,
                    hemorrhage,
                    multiple gestation

*D/C if maternal HR > 140, FHR > 180,
maternal BP < 90/60, CP, VPB's, PSVT or
atrial fibrillation
*Monitor for ↑ blood glucose, pulmonary
edema, RV failure

Antidote: propranolol 0.5 – 1.0 mg slow IV or
           verapamil 5 – 10 mg slow IV
- -

THEOPHYLLINE (Slo-Phyllin)
Use: Parentral theophylline for patients not
currently receiving theophylline

Dose: Load: 4.7 mg/kg IV slowly; then
              maintenance infusion
              *MAX rate of injection:
              20 mg/min

Adult (nonsmoker):
-       0.55 mg/kg/hr IV × 12 hr, then
        0.39 mg/kg/hr

Otherwise healthy adult smokers:
-       0.79 mg/kg/hr IV × 12 hr, then
        0.63 mg/kg/hr

                        (con't)

183

Medications – Theophylline (con't)
Older adult w/ cor pulmonale:
- 0.47 mg/kg/hr IV × 12 hr, then 0.24 mg/kg/hr

Adults w/ CHF or liver dz:
- 0.39 mg/kg/hr IV × 12 hr, then 0.08 – 0.16 mg/kg/hr

Children 9 – 16 yo:
- 0.79 mg/kg/hr IV × 12 hr, then 0.63 mg/kg/hr

Children 6 mo – 9 yo:
- 0.95 mg/kg/hr IV × 12 hr, then 0.79 mg/kg/hr

Neonatal Apnea:
- Load 5 mg/kg PO × 1
- Maintenance 3 – 6 mg/kg/d PO ÷ q 6 – 8 hr

*Therapeutic levels
- Asthma: 10 – 20 mg/L
- Apnea: 7 – 13 mg/L

Use: Oral and parentral theophylline for acute
bronchospasm in patients currently
receiving theophylline

Dose: Adult/Child: each 0.5 mg/kg IV or PO
(loading dose) will ↑
plasma levels by 1 μg/ml.
Base dose on serum
theophylline level.

- -

THIOPENTAL (Pentothal)
Use: Anesthesia induction, barbiturate
coma

Dose: Adult/Child: 2 – 6 mg/kg

Maintenance: 5 – 15 mg/kg/hr titrated to EEG

Use: Cerebral edema

Dose: Adult/Child: 1.5 – 5.0 mg/kg IV
*MR PRN for ↑ ICP

Contraindication: Acute intermittent porphyria

- -

TIROFIBAN (Aggrastat)

Use: Acute coronary syndrome
*GPIIb/IIIa receptor antagonist

Dose: Adult: Start 0.4 μg/kg/min × 30 min,
then ↓ to 0.1 μg/kg/min ×
48 – 108 hr or until 12 – 24 hr
after coronary intervention

Contraindications:
- Active internal bleeding
- Hemorrhagic CVA or CVA
- Bleeding diathesis
- Concomitant parentral use of other
  GPIIb/IIIa receptor antagonists
- Recent (within 6 weeks) major surgery or
  trauma
- Intracranial neoplasm, AVM or aneurysm
- Severe uncontrolled HTN
- Aortic dissection
- Acute pericarditis
- History of thrombocytopenia after
  previous tirofiban therapy

*Use w/ heparin to keep PTT twice nml
*Use ½ dose w/ CrCl < 30 ml/min
- -

TISSUE PLASMINOGEN ACTIVATOR (tPA, Alteplase)

Use: Thrombolytic

Dose: Adult (Front-loading regimen for AMI):
- 15 mg over 2 min
- 0.75 mg/kg over 30 min
  (not to exceed 50 mg)
- 0.50 mg/kg over 60 min
  (not to exceed 35 mg)
  *MAX DOSE: ≤ 100 mg

Dose: Adult (Acute Ischemic CVA):
- 0.9 mg/kg IV infusion over 1 hr
  w/ 10% of the total dose
  administered as an initial IV
  bolus over 1 min
  *MAX DOSE: 90 mg
  *Must be given within 3 hr after
  sx **occur** and an intracranial
  bleed has been ruled out

Dose: Adult (Acute Pulmonary Embolism):
- 50 – 100 mg IV infusion over
  2 – 6 hr
  *Not clinically agreed upon as
  to proper dose and time
  frame for administration

(con't)

Medications – tPA (con't)

Contraindications:
- Active internal bleeding or known bleeding diathesis
- History of CVA
- Intracranial or intraspinal surgery or trauma within 2 months
- Intracranial neoplasm, AVM, aneurysm
- Known bleeding diathesis
- Severe uncontrolled HTN

*tPA converts fibrin bound plasminogen to plasmin
*Antidote is aminocaproic acid – use only if uncontrolled hemorrhage

- - - - - - - - - - - - - - - - - - - -

TROMETHAMINE (THAM)

Use: Correction of metabolic acidosis

Dose: Adult/Infant/Child:
  *Depends on base deficit

- When deficit is known:

tromethamine ml (0.3 M sol'n) = kg wt $\times$ base deficit (mEq/L)

-   When deficit is NOT known

    3.5 – 6.0 ml/kg/dose IV
    (1 – 2 mEq/kg/dose)
    MAX: 500 mg/kg/dose

Use: Correction of excess acidity of stored
blood preserved w/ acid citrate dextrose
(ACD)

Dose: 14 – 70 ml of 0.3 M sol'n added to each
500 ml of blood

Contraindications: Uremia, anuria, chronic
respiratory acidosis

SE: Cardiovascular venospasm,
hyperkalemia, hypoglycemia, necrosis w/
extravasation, respiratory depression,
hemorrhagic hepatic necrosis (when
administered through umbilical vein)

*↓ dose w/ renal impairment and monitor pH
carefully
- -

VALPROIC ACID (Depacon)

Use: Seizures, status epilepticus

Dose: Adult/Child: 10 – 15 mg/kg IV
MAX: 60 mg/kg/d

SE: Sedation, N/V, pancreatitis,
thrombocytopenia, elevated liver
enzymes, toxic hepatitis, alopecia

- - - - - - - - - - - - - - - - - - - -

VASOPRESSIN (Pitressin)

Use: GI hemorrhage

Dose: Adult: Start @ 0.2 – 0.4 U/min
*↑ dose PRN to MAX DOSE of
1 U/min
*Mix: 100 U in 250 ml
(concentration 0.4 U/ml)

Child: Start @ 0.002 – 0.005 U/kg/min
*↑ dose PRN to 0.1 U/kg/min

SE: Myocardial ischemia, MI, ventricular
arrhythmias, cardiac arrest, mesenteric
ischemia or infarction, cutaneous
ischemic necrosis

*Once bleeding is controlled gradually ↓ rate
*Use w/ extreme caution in patients w/ vascular or cardiovascular dz
*Concomitant IV infusion of nitroglycerin may ↓ undesirable cardiovascular side effects

- - - - - - - - - - - - - - - - - - - -

VECURONIUM (Norcuron)

Use: Nondepolarizing neuromuscular blocker

Dose: Adult/Infant > 2 mo: 0.08 – 0.1 mg/kg IV

      Maintenance: 0.05 – 0.1 mg/kg IV
              q 1 hr PRN

      Continuous IV: 0.8 – 1.2 mg/kg/hr for
              ages > 1 yr to adult

Dose: Neonates: 0.1 mg/kg IV

      Maintenance: 0.03 – 0.15 mg/kg IV q
              1 – 2 hr PRN

Duration: 25 – 40 min

*Reversed w/ neostigmine or edrophonium

Use: Defasciculating dose before succinylcholine

Dose: 0.04 – 0.06 mg/kg

- - - - - - - - - - - - - - - - - - - -

VERAPAMIL (Calan)

Use: Ca^{++} channel blocker for atrial fibrillation, PSVT

Dose: Adult: 5 – 10 mg slow IV (0.15 mg/kg)

1 – 15 yo: 0.1 – 0.3 mg/kg slow IV
MAX DOSE: 5 mg 1st dose,
10 mg 2nd dose

0 – 1 yo: 0.1 – 0.2 mg/kg

Contraindications: Atrial flutter/fibrillation w/
accessory bypass tract,
patients receiving IV
β-blockers, VT, sick sinus
syndrome, 2° or 3° AVB
w/o pacemaker, LV
dysfunction

*Give over 2 – 3 min
*MR × 1 q 30 min for all doses
*Can cause apnea in neonates
*Can cause paralytic ileus
*↑ digoxin level
*Hypotension is due to vasodilation – can ↓
hypotensive effect if the patient is pretreated
w/ 10 ml of 10% Ca^{++} gluconate

- -

NEUROLOGY

CRANIAL NERVES

I	Smell
II	Vision, Marcus-Gunn pupil
III	Parasympathetic – pupillary constriction from the Edinger-Westphal nucleus Sympathetic – pupillary dilation, eyelid elevation
III, IV, VI	Extra-ocular motions
V	Facial sensation

V_1: Opthalmic – corneal reflex
V_2: Maxillary
V_3: Mandibular
Motor – muscles of mastication, jaw clenching. Lateral jaw movement (R pterygoid contraction moves the jaw L). Pterygoid also controls protrusion and retraction of jaw.

VII	Facial movement, motor of corneal reflex, (+) forehead wrinkle = upper motor neuron lesion; (–) forehead wrinkle = lower motor neuron lesion aka CN VII palsy (Bell's Palsy).
VIII	Vestibular branch – hearing Cochlear branch – balance
IX	Sensory – gag Motor – swallowing, elevate palate *Uvula deviates away from lesion
X	Motor – gag, swallow, uvula elevation, cough, phonation – "K"

(con't)

Cranial Nerves (con't)

XI   Shoulder shrug – trapezius;
               head turn – sternocleidomastoid

XII   Speech – "L", "T", "D", "N". Push
               tongue against cheek, stick tongue
               out. Upper motor neuron lesion –
               tongue deviates to opposite side of
               lesion. Lower motor neuron lesion –
               tongue deviates to side of lesion.

CRANIAL NERVE LOCATIONS:
II, III, IV – midbrain
V – pons
VI, VII, VIII – pontomedullary junction
IX, X, XI, XII – medulla

```
                 Superior      Inferior
                 Rectus III    Oblique III
                     ↑             ↑
Lateral                                        Medial
Rectus VI  ←————————  ●  ————————→  Rectus III
                     ↓             ↓
                 Inferior      Superior
                 Rectus III    Oblique IV
```

● = pupil
*Depiction of right eye

Weber Test: Place the tuning fork in the
             midline @ the vertex of the
             patient's head. The patient
             should hear the sound equally in
             both ears.
-   Conduction loss is present if the patient
    hears the tuning fork louder in the
    abnormal ear.
-   Sensory neural loss is present if the
    patient hears the tuning fork louder in the
    normal ear.

Rinné Test: Place the tuning fork on the
             patient's mastoid process and
             count the time it takes until the
             patient no longer hears the
             sound. Quickly bring the tuning
             fork in front of the patient's ear
             and count the time it takes until
             the patient can no longer hear the
             sound. Air conduction (AC)
             should be twice that of bone
             conduction (BC).
-   If BC > AC = conductive hearing loss on
    the affected side
-   If AC > BC or AC = BC, then it is a
    sensorineural hearing loss
*The results only correlate w/ abnormal
  hearing

- -

DERMATOMES

Back of Head	C_2
Clavicle	C_4
Arms	$C_5 - T_2$
1st Digit (thumb)	C_6
3rd Digit	C_7
5th Digit	C_8
Nipple Line	T_4
Xiphoid Process	T_7
Umbilicus	T_{10}
Inguinal Crease	L_1
Anterior Surface Thigh	L_3
Medial Side of Foot	L_4
Dorsum of Foot	L_5
Great Toe	L_5
Lateral Side of Foot	S_1
Sole of Foot	S_1
Perineum	$S_3 - S_5$
Anus	S_5

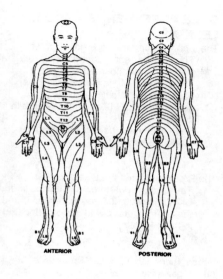

ANTERIOR POSTERIOR

(From *The Mont Reid Surgical Handbook*, 4th ed, St. Louis, 1997, Mosby)

— — — — — — — — — — — — — — — — — —

197

GAZE PREFERENCE – FOCAL LESIONS

The L cortex controls the R gaze center
- The R gaze center controls the ipsilateral CN VI nucleus (located in the pons)
- The CN VI nucleus is controlling the lateral rectus muscle and the contralateral CN III nucleus (located in the midbrain)
- The CN III nucleus is controlling the medial rectus muscle

The R cortex control the L gaze center
- The L gaze center controls the ipsilateral CN VI nucleus (located in the pons) and the contralateral CN III nucleus (located in the midbrain)

If the patient has a R Gaze Preference (aka L gaze palsy) the lesion is a(n):
1. Destructive lesion located in the R cortex OR
2. Destructive lesion located in the L pons OR
3. Irritative lesion in the L cortex

If the patient has a L Gaze Preference
(aka R gaze palsy) the lesion is a(n):
1. Destructive lesion located in the L cortex
   OR
2. Destructive lesion located in the R pons
   OR
3. Irritative lesion located in the R cortex
- -

HERNIATION SYNDROMES

Cushing's Reflex: Late finding of ↑ ICP
- ↑ BP
- ↓ HR
- Irregular respirations

- Falx cerebri: separates the two cerebral
  hemispheres vertically
  down to the brainstem

- Tentorium cerebelli: separates the
  cerebellum and
  brainstem from the
  cerebrum at the
  base of the skull

(con't)

199

Uncal Herniation:
- Most common
- Uncus of the temporal lobe is displaced inferiorly through the medial edge of the tentorium
- Lesion located in the temporal lobe or lateral middle fossa

S/S
- Ipsilateral fixed and dilated pupil (can also be contralateral to injury)
- Contralateral paralysis (can also be ipsilateral to the injury)

Central Transtentorial:
- Cerebrum is pushed down onto the midbrain causing the midbrain to compress the brainstem which causes herniation of the brainstem through the foramen magnum
- Lesion located midline in the frontal or occipital lobes

S/S
- Initially
    - Bilateral pinpoint pupils
    - Bilateral Babinski's sign
    - ↑ muscle tone
- Later
    - Fixed and midpoint pupils
    - Prolonged hyperventilation
    - Decorticate posturing

Cerebellotonsillar:
- Cerebellar tonsils herniate through the foramen magnum

S/S
- Pinpoint pupils
- Flaccid paralysis
- Sudden death

Upward Transtentorial:
- Lesion located in the posterior fossa

S/S
- Pinpoint pupils
- Conjugate downward gaze
- Absence of vertical eye movement
- Sudden death

GOALS:
- Maintain MAP $\geq$ 90 mmHg
  *SBP 120 – 140 mmHg
- Maintain CPP $\geq$ 70 mmHg
  *CPP = MAP – ICP
  *Autoregulation is maintained when CPP is between 50 – 150 mmHg
- Maintain ICP $\leq$ 20 – 25 mmHg
  *wnl ICP = 0 – 10 mmHg

(con't)

Herniation Syndromes (con't)

Tx:

- ABC's w/ c-spine control if needed
- Rapid sequence intubation
- Elevate HOB 30° if permissible
- Maintain PaO_2 > 60 mmHg
- Maintain MAP ≥ 90 mmHg
  - *Vasopressors may be harmful, however, they may be used w/ ↓ BP if the hypotension is not caused from volume loss
  - *Norepinephrine and/or phenylephrine are preferred
- Maintain Hct > 30%
- Hyperventilate to maintain $PaCO_2$ 25 – 30 mmHg
  - *Use ONLY for documented ↑ ICP
    - Unilateral dilated pupil
    - ↓ LOC
    - Posturing
  - *Causes cerebral vasoconstriction within 30 sec leading to ↓ ICP
  - *Short-term therapy only
- Mannitol 0.25 – 1.0 g/kg IV
  - *Effects seen within 30 min and last 6 – 8 hrs

*If HTN exists independently from the ↑ ICP, lower the MAP no > 30% from the systemic blood pressure – nitroprusside is preferred

- -

HERNIATION RESPIRATORY PATTERNS

Cheyne-Stokes: Involvement of the diencephalon above the thalamus

Midbrain: Central neurogenic hyperventilation

Upper Pons: Apneustic respirations

Lower Pons: Cluster respirations

Medulla: Ataxic respirations

- -

LOC – ALTERED

A alcohol
E epilepsy, encephalitis
I infection, ↑ ICP
O overdose, poison, opiates
U uremia

T trauma, temperature, tumor
I insulin
P psychogenic
S shock, stroke, syncope, sz

- -

LUMBAR PUNCTURE/
CSF VALUES

Perform LP @ L_{4-5} in adult and @ L_{4-5} or $L_5 - S_1$ in infant

Queckenstedt's Test: May indicate chronic adhesive arachnoiditis from SAH, meningitis, intrathecal PCN, spinal anesthetics (certain forms), trauma, surgery or radiologic contrast material.

- Perform LP, have a second person compress the jugular vein. Normal physiologic response is to see a rise in CSF pressure on the manometer. If there is a blocked spinal canal, no transmission of pressure through the CSF occurs and no increase on the manometer is seen. If (+), gather more information or tests from the patient.

Tube #1: Protein, glucose, lactate
Tube #2: Gram stain, C&S
Tube #3: Cell count w/ differential
Tube #4: Hold for additional studies

CSF VALUES:

Volume

Adult: 90 – 150 ml
Child: 60 – 100 ml

Clarity

Crystal clear, colorless

Pressure 75 – 150 mmH$_2$O
*To convert cmH$_2$O to mmHg: cmH$_2$O/13.6 = mmHg

Total Cell Count 0 – 5 WBC/µl
*Normally all cells are lymphocytes
*No PMN's or RBC's should be observed
*If traumatic LP subtract 1 WBC / 700 RBC's

*Prior antibiotics ∅ alter total CSF WBC's, glucose or percent of patients w/ a (+) CIE or latex agglutination test
*Prior antibiotics will ↓ CSF protein and ↓ possibility of seeing bacteria on gram stain

Specific Gravity 1.006 – 1.008
Osmolality 280 – 290 mOsm/kg

Albumin : Globulin Ratio 8:1
Bilirubin 0
Calcium 2.1 – 2.7 mEq/L
Chloride 118 – 132 mEq/L
Cholesterol 0.2 – 0.6 mg/dl
CO$_2$ Content 25 – 30 mEq/L
Creatinine 0.5 – 1.2 mg/dl
Glucose 40 – 70 mg/dl

(con't)

205

Lumbar Puncture/CSF Values (con't)

Glutamine	6 – 15 mg/dl
Lactic Acid	24 mg/dl
LDH	1/10 that of serum
Magnesium	2.4 mEq/L
PCO_2	42 – 53 mmHg
pH	7.30 – 7.40
PO_2	40 – 44 mmHg
Potassium	2.0 – 3.5 mEq/L
Protein	15 – 45 mg/dl (lumbar)
	15 – 25 mg/dl (cisternal)
	5 – 15 mg/dl (ventricular)

*If traumatic LP subtract 1 mg Pr⁻ / 1000 RBCs'

Sodium	144 – 154 mEq/L
Urea Nitrogen	6 – 16 mg/dl
Uric Acid	0.5 – 4.5 mg/dl
VDRL	Negative

- - - - - - - - - - - - - - - - - - - -

MENINGEAL IRRITATION

Brudzinski's Sign: (+) sign: patient flexes the lower limbs on passive flexion of the head to the chest

Kernig's Sign: (+) sign: pain and resistance on extending the patients leg at the knee after flexing the thigh on the body
*May be unilateral or bilateral

Nuchal Rigidity: neck resistance to flexion
*Appears @ 18 mo or older

HA: frontally or occipitally localized. May
extend down the neck. ↑ w/ sudden
movement or w/ forceful cough.

- -

MYOTOMES

Abduct Arm	C_5
Adduct Arm	$C_6 - C_8$
Flex Elbow	$C_5 - C_6$
Extend Elbow	$C_7 - C_8$
Pronate/Supinate	C_6
Wrist Extension	C_6
Wrist Flexion	C_7
Finger Extension	C_7
Finger Flexion	C_8
Finger Adduct/Abduct	T_1
Flex/Adduct/Med. Rotate Hip	$L_1 - L_3$
Extend Knee	$L_3 - L_4$
Dorsiflex/Invert Ankle	$L_4 - L_5$
Evert Ankle	$L_5 - S_1$
Plantar Flexion	$S_1 - S_2$

- -

NEUROLOGICAL TESTS
Cerebellar Testing
- Romberg (eyes closed): proprioceptive loss secondary to peripheral neuropathology or spinal cord dorsal column neuropathology
- Finger-to-Nose (eyes closed): sensory ataxia
- Finger-to-Finger (eyes open): sensory ataxia
- Rapid Rhythmic Alternating Movements: finger tap, diadokokinesia, hand or foot tapping
- Heel to Toe Walking

Corneal Reflex

Stimulus	OD	OS	Anatomy of Defect
OD	+	+	Brainstem intact
OD	+	−	L efferent lesion
OD	−	+	R efferent lesion
OD	−	−	Further testing indicated – could be R afferent lesions, bilateral efferent or afferent lesion

Deep Tendon Reflex Grading

Grade	DTR Response
0	No response
1+	Sluggish or diminished
2+	Active or expected response
3+	More brisk than expected, slightly hyperactive
4+	Brisk, hyperactive, w/ intermittent or transient clonus

Motor System Grading

5 = Active motion against full resistance (Normal)
4 = Active motion against some resistance (Good)
3 = Active motion against gravity (Fair)
2 = Active motion w/ gravity eliminated (Poor)
1 = Barely detectable motion (Trace)
0 = No motion or muscular contraction detected (None)
*Test strength in upper and lower extremities, proximally and distally

Oculocepahlic Reflex (Doll's Eyes)

Cortex Intact	Brainstem Intact	Reflex Elicited
−	−	−
−	+	+
+	−	−
+	+	−

(con't)

Neurological Test (con't)
Oculovestibular Response
(Cold Caloric Test)

Cortex Intact	Brainstem Intact	Tonic Component	Quick Component
−	−	−	−
−	+	+	−
+	−	−	−
+	+	+	+

*Have the patient's HOB 30°, use 30 ml cold H₂O and instill over 30 sec, repeat × 3
*If the patient is unconscious, the fast component will be lost. The fast component is from the cortex while the slow component is from the brainstem.
*If eye movement is up, down or squewed it indicates partial brainstem functioning
*COWS: cold opposite, warm same w/ regard to the fast component

Posturing
Elicited by noxious stimuli

Decorticate: Flexion of the arms @ the elbow, adduction @ the shoulder, extension of the legs @ the ankle
- Occurs when a lesion involves the cerebral hemispheres or internal capsule

- Usually involves the thalamus directly or a large hemispheric mass compressing the thalamus from above

Decerebrate: Extension @ the elbow, internal rotation of the shoulder and forearm and leg extension
- Occurs when a lesion is located in the midbrain, brainstem or pons
- Indicates more severe brain damage due to a lower lesion

Flaccid: Lesion of the lower medulla

*Bilateral symmetric posturing may be seen w/ structural or metabolic disorders
*Unilateral or asymmetric posturing is suggestive of structural dz in the contralateral cerebral hemisphere or brain stem
*Patients w/ pontine and medullary lesions usually ∅ respond to pain but may show some knee flexion

- -

PUPIL GAUGE - mm

2   3   4   5   6   7   8   9

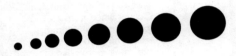

PUPILLARY RESPONSES

Diencephalon involvement:
- Small reactive pupils w/ very bright light
- Sympathetics are not working
- Injury to hypothalamus or above

Midbrain Tectal (Dorsal):
- Large, fixed pupils that vary in size spontaneously w/o light stimulus

Midbrain Tegmentum (Ventral):
- Midsize, fixed pupils
- Autonomics not functioning

Pons involvement:
- Small, reactive pupils, possibly pinpoint
- Sympathetics not functioning

CN III (Uncal Herniation):
- Ipsilateral dilated, fixed pupil
- Parasympathetics not functioning on involved side

- -

REFLEXES
Deep Tendon Reflexes

Biceps Brachii	$C_5 - C_6$
Brachioradialis	$C_6 - C_7$
Triceps Brachii	$C_6 - C_8$
Patellar	$L_2 - L_4$
Achilles	$S_1 - S_2$

Superficial Reflexes

Upper Abdominal	$T_7 - T_9$
Lower Abdominal	$T_{10} - T_{11}$
Cremasteric	$T_{12} - L_2$
Plantar	$L_4 - S_2$

- -

SEIZURE LOCATION AND ASSOCIATED SYMPTOMS

Frontal Cortex: psychic sx, no focal sx, adversive turning of head

Motor Cortex: clonic movements

Parietal Cortex: paresthesias

Occipital Cortex: uniformed visual hallucinations

Temporal Cortex:
- Anterior Temporal: psychic sx, déjà vu, automatisms

- Sylvian: epigastric sensations, movement of mouth or face, dreamy state, automatisms, hallucinations of taste

- Mid Temporal: auditory hallucinations, vertigo, depression, déjà vu, depersonalization

- Posterior Temporal: complex visual hallucinations, dreamy state, depression

Medial Surface: automatisms, psychic sx,
olfactory hallucinations

Uncal Gyrus: olfactory hallucinations: usually
foul smelling

- - - - - - - - - - - - - - - - - - - -

SEIZURE MEDICATIONS
Diazepam (Valium)
Dose: Adult: 5 – 10 mg IV q 10 – 15 min
MAX TOTAL DOSE: 30 mg

Child > 1 mo: 0.2 – 0.5 mg/kg IV
q 15 – 30 min
MAX TOTAL DOSE:
< 5 yo: 5 mg
≥ 5 yo: 10 mg

Neonate: 0.3 – 0.75 mg/kg IV q
15 – 30 min × 2 – 3 doses

*Stops the convulsion but it may not stop
the brain seizure activity

(con't)

Seizure Medications (con't)
FOSPHENYTOIN (Cerebyx)
*All dosing is expressed as phenytoin
 sodium equivalents (PE)

Dose: Adult: 15 – 20 mg PE/kg IV

      Maintenance: 4 – 6 mg PE/kg/d IV/IM

*∅ administer at a rate > 150 mg PE/min

Glucose 25%
Dose: Peds: 2 – 4 ml/kg (0.5 – 1.0 g/kg) sol'n
             × 1 dose
         *Consider using if cause of sz is
         obscure

Lorazepam (Ativan)
Dose: Adult: 2 – 4 mg slow IV over 2 – 5 min
         MR in 5 – 15 min
         MAX DOSE: 8 mg in 12 hr

      Child/Infant/Neonate: 0.05 – 0.1 mg/kg
                  slow IV over
                  2 – 5 min
                  MR 0.05 mg/kg ×
                  1 in 10 – 15 min

Pentobarbital (Nembutal)
For barbiturate coma

Dose: Adult/Child: Load: 10 – 15 mg/kg IV
over 1 – 2 hr

Maintenance: 1 – 3
mg/kg/hr

*Therapeutic serum level: 20 – 40 mg/L

Phenobarbital (Luminal)
Dose: Adult: 10 – 20 mg/kg IV slowly
MAX TOTAL: 600 mg

Maintentance: 60 mg IV q 3 hr

Child/Infant/Neonate: 15 – 20 mg in
single or ÷ dose.
May give
additional
5 mg/kg
q 15 – 30 min.
MAX TOTAL:
30 mg/kg

(con't)

217

Seizure Meds – Phenobarbital (con't)
     Maintenance:
-   > 12 yo: 1 – 3 mg/kg/d ÷
        qd – BID
-   6 – 12 yo: 4 – 6 mg/kg/d ÷
        qd – BID
-   1 – 5 yo: 6 – 8 mg/kg/d ÷
        qd – BID
-   Neonates: 3 – 5 mg/kg/d ÷
        qd – BID

*Give slow IVP, no faster than 1 mg/kg/min

Phenytoin (Dilantin)
Dose: Adult: 10 – 15 mg/kg IV
        MAX TOTAL: 1.5 g
        *∅ exceed 50 mg/min

     Maintenance: 100 mg IV/PO q
        6 – 8 hr

(desired – measured) × kg wt × 0.8 = mg dose
to give if patient levels are low

     Child: 15 – 20 mg/kg IV
        *∅ exceed 1 mg/kg/min in infants
        *∅ exceed 50 mg/min in children

Neonate: Start w/ 5 mg/kg/d IV/PO
÷ q 12 hr
*Usual range is 5 – 8 mg/kg/d
÷ q 8 – 12 hr
*∅ exceed 0.5 mg/kg/min in
neonates

*For IV extravasation use lidocaine,
nitroglycerin paste or regitine
*NOT compatible w/ D_5W, use 0.9% NS

Thiopental (Pentothal)
For barbiturate coma

Dose: Adult/Child: 2 – 6 mg/kg

Maintenance: 5 – 15 mg/kg/hr titrated to EEG

Valproic Acid (Depacon)

Dose: Adult/Child: 10 – 15 mg/kg IV
MAX: 60 mg/kg/d
- -

SPINAL TRACTS – TESTING INDIVIDUAL

Spinal Tracts	Neurological Tests
Ascending Tracts	
Lateral Spinothalamic	Superficial pain Temperature
Anterior Spinothalamic	Superficial touch Deep pressure
Posterior Column	Vibration Deep pressure Position sense Stereognosis Point location Two-point discrimination
Anterior and Dorsal Spinocerebellar	Proprioception

Descending Tracts

Lateral and Anterior Corticospinal	Rapid rhythmic alternating movements Voluntary movement DTR's Plantar reflex
Medial and Lateral Reticulospinal	Posture and Romberg Gait Instinctual reactions

Minimal Distances of Two-point Discrimination

Body Part	Minimal Distance (mm)
Tongue	1
Fingertips	2 – 8
Toes	3 – 8
Palms of hands	8 – 12
Chest and forearms	40
Back	40 – 70
Upper arms and thighs	75

- -

STROKE PATIENT – ACUTE GENERAL MANAGEMENT

1.	IV fluids	Avoid D_5W and excessive fluid loading
2.	Blood sugar	Determine immediately and administer a bolus of $D_{50}W$ if the patient is hypoglycemic or administer insulin if the patient's blood glucose is > 300 mg/dl
3.	Thiamine	100 mg IV if the patient is Malnourished or an alcoholic
4.	Oxygen	Pulse oximetry and supplement O_2 as needed
5.	Febrile	Administer acetaminophen
6.	NPO	If the patient is at risk for aspiration

- - - - - - - - - - - - - - - - - - - -

STROKE SCALE – CINCINNATI PREHOSPITAL

Facial Droop
- Have patient show their teeth or smile

- Normal – both sides of face move equally
- Abnormal – one side of face does not move as well as the other side

Arm Drift
- Patient closes their eyes and holds both of their arms out w/ palms up

- Normal – both arms move the same *or* both arms do no move at all (other findings, such as pronator grip, may be helpful)
- Abnormal – one arm does not move *or* one arm drifts down compared w/ the other

Speech
- Have the patient say, "You can't teach an old dog new tricks."

- Normal – patient uses correct words w/ no slurring
- Abnormal – patient slurs words, uses inappropriate words, *or* is unable to speak

- -

SUBARACHNOID HEMORRHAGE – HUNT AND HESS SCALE

Grade	Neurological Status
I	Asymptomatic or minimal headache
II	Moderate to severe headache or nuchal rigidity – no neurological deficit except cranial nerve palsy
III	Drowsy or confusion – minimal focal neurological deficit
IV	Stuporous – moderate to severe hemiparesis
V	Deep coma – decerebrate posturing

*Nimodipine (Nimotop) 60 mg q 4 hr × 21 d for grade I – III. Peak effect: 1 hr. Will ↓ BP.

- -

THROMBOLYTIC THERAPY CHECKLIST – ACUTE ISCHEMIC STROKE

Inclusion Criteria (all YES boxes must be checked before treatment)

YES

☐ Age 18 years or older
☐ Clinical diagnosis of ischemic stroke causing measurable neurological deficit
☐ Symptom **onset** < 180 min before treatment would begin

Exclusion Criteria (all NO boxes must be checked before treatment)

NO

- ❑ Evidence of intracranial hemorrhage on noncontrast head CT
- ❑ Only minor or rapidly improving stroke symptoms
- ❑ High clinical suspicion of subarachnoid hemorrhage even w/ normal CT
- ❑ Active internal bleeding (e.g. GI bleeding or urinary bleeding within last 21 days)
- ❑ Known bleeding diathesis, including but not limited to:
  - Platelet count < 100,000/mm^3
  - Patient has received heparin within 48 hr and had an ↑ aPTT (> upper limit of wnl for laboratory)
  - Recent use of anticoagulant (e.g. warfarin) and ↑ PT > 15 seconds
- ❑ Within 3 months of intracranial surgery, serious head trauma, or previous stroke
- ❑ Within 14 days of major surgery or serious trauma
- ❑ Recent arterial puncture @ noncompressible site
- ❑ Lumbar puncture within 7 days
- ❑ History of intracranial hemorrhage, arteriovenous malformation, or aneurysm
- ❑ Witnessed seizure @ stroke onset
- ❑ Recent acute MI
- ❑ On repeated measurements, SBP > 185 mmHg or DBP > 110 mmHg @ time of treatment, requiring aggressive treatment to ↓ BP to within these limits

- - - - - - - - - - - - - - - - - - -

VISUAL FIELD DEFECTS

Central Scotoma:
- Inflammation of optic disk or nerve

Unilateral Blindness:
- Complete lesion of optic nerve

Bitemporal Hemianopia:
- Pressure exerted on optic chiasm possibly from pituitary tumor

Unilateral Nasal Hemianopia:
- Perichiasmal lesion

Homonymous Hemianopia:
- Lesion of optic tract, a complete lesion of the optic radiation, posterior cerebral artery occlusion

Homonymous Superior Quadrantanopia:
- Partial involvement of the optic radiation by a lesion in the temporal lobe (Meyer's Loop)

Homonymous Inferior Quadrantanopia:
- Partial involvement of the optic radiation by a lesion in the parietal lobe

Homonymous Hemianopia w/ Macular Sparing:
- Posterior cerebral artery occlusion

- -

ABRUPTIO PLACENTA

Dark red vaginal bleeding, sometimes w/o external signs of hemorrhage, due to separation of placenta after 20+ weeks gestation

- Significant fetal and maternal mortality
- ↑ incidence associated w/ HTN, pre-eclampsia, trauma – especially MVA's
- 80% of all cases occur before the onset of labor

S/S: Constant abdominal pain, uterine tenderness between contractions, tetanic uterine contractions, ↑ uterine tone, bleeding (may be concealed), **shock, DIC**

- Monitor for DIC w/ wall clot test: Place 5 ml blood in red top tube, place upright. If a clot does not form within 6 – 12 min or if clot lysis occurs within 30 min an abnormality in clotting may be present.
  *Can be used if lab is not available

Tx: DIC/shock:
- 100% O$_2$/NRB
- 2 large bore IV's on blood tubing
- Administer blood or SPA 25% (50 – 100 ml, MR in 15 – 30 min)
- Elevate feet, MAST – inflate legs only
- Consider ephedrine 25 mg slow IV
- Prepare for emergency c-section

- - - - - - - - - - - - - - - - - - - -

AMNIOTIC FLUID EMBOLISM

Amniotic fluid enters maternal circulation resulting in obstruction of the pulmonary vasculature usually after a tumultuous delivery. Mortality rate > 90%.

Complications: DIC, uterine atony, hemorrhage, acute cor pulmonale, R heart failure, pulmonary edema

S/S: Sudden acute dyspnea, cyanosis, shock, CP, cough, pulmonary edema, sz

Tx:
- O_2/NRB, intubate PRN
- Crystalloids/colloids for hypotension
- FHT monitoring

If the patient delivered:
- Oxytocin 20 – 40 U in 1000 ml LR @ 150 – 250 ml/hr
- Fundal massage @ least q 15 min
- Morphine 2 – 5 mg over 1 – 2 min

- -

CERVICAL DILATION

- Diameter in cm @ internal os
- Expressed from 0 (closed) to
  10 cm (complete) dilation

One finger (snug)   = 1 cm
One finger (loose) = 2 cm
Two fingers (snug) = 3 cm
Two fingers (loose) = 4 cm
> 5 cm is estimated

- -

DELIVERY, EMERGENCY

Can be expected when the perineum bulges
and the fetal scalp is visible at the introitus

POSITIONING

Lateral Sims:
- Slower descent
- Less tension on the perineal tissue
- May allow delivery w/o an episiotomy

Dorsal Lithotomy:
- Better visualization
- Better manual control of the delivery
  process

(con't)

Delivery, Emergency – Dorsal Lithotomy Position (con't)

- Easier to perform episiotomy
  *If this position is chosen, tilt the mother to one side to avoid vena caval compression
  *Mother should be at the edge of the bed or her pelvis raised on pillows to allow adequate room for delivery of the baby's head and shoulders

PROCEDURE
Delivery of the Head
- Manually, gently stretch the perineum
- Perform episiotomy if needed
  - Inject 5 – 10 ml of 1% lidocaine w/ a small gauge needle
  - If lidocaine is unavailable, the episiotomy can be performed w/ minimal pain when the perineum is fully stretched
- As the head emerges, place the palm of one hand over the head to assist w/ wnl head extension
- Control the descent of the head to avoid rapid expulsion
- **ASK THE MOTHER NOT TO PUSH**
  - Have the mother pant or breathe through her nose
- Drape the other hand w/ a sterile cloth
- Gently lift the baby's chin posterior toward the maternal anus

- At this point the baby should extend further and rotate
- Immediately palpate the baby's neck for a nuchal cord
    - If present and loose, gently slip it over the baby's head
    - If present and tight, clamp the cord in two places and cut the cord between the clamps
- Wipe the baby's face and suction the **mouth** first, then the nose

Delivery of the Shoulders
- Place both hands on either side of the baby's head and apply gentle downward traction to ease the anterior shoulder under the pubic symphysis
    - If resistance, have an assistant apply **suprapubic** pressure
- Once the anterior shoulder is visible, gently apply upward traction to deliver the posterior shoulder
- Be sure to support the baby's head w/ the posterior hand

(con't)

Delivery, Emergency (con't)
Delivery of the Body and Legs
- Slide the anterior hand along the baby's back
- Place the index finger between the lower legs and grasp the baby's legs w/ the thumb and third finger
- ∅ **hold the baby upside down**
- Cradle the baby w/ the same arm that is grasping the legs
- Clamp the cord in two places and cut the cord between the two clamps

SHOULDER DYSTOCIA
- Impaction of the anterior shoulder behind the pubic symphysis
- **TIME is of the essence!**
- Recognized when mild downward traction fails to deliver the shoulder
- The fetal head will be tight against the perineum – Turtle Sign

POSITIONING – SHOULDER DYSTOCIA
- Place the mother's perineum at the end of the bed
- Sharply flex the mother's legs toward the abdomen – McRoberts maneuver
- Perform a generous episiotomy
  *Extend through the anal sphincter if necessary

232

- Apply **suprapubic** pressure to deliver the anterior shoulder
- If these measures fail
  - Rotate one or both shoulders toward the baby's chest

    OR

  - Progressively rotate the posterior shoulder 180° while an assistant applies **suprapubic** pressure at a 45° angle in the same direction of the rotated shoulder to allow release of the impacted anterior shoulder

- If these measures fail
  - Attempt to deliver the posterior arm by grasping the forearm, which is still in the uterus, and raising it above the baby's head out through the introitus

- Should this fail
  - Fracture the anterior clavicle or humerus and deliver the baby

(con't)

Delivery, Emergency (con't)
POSTPARTUM
- Allow the placenta to separate spontaneously
    - A gush of blood and lengthening of the cord herald placental delivery
- Once the placenta is delivered, massage the uterus to aid in contraction
- Start an oxytocin gtt
- If excessive bleeding
    - Vigorous uterine massage
    - ↑ IV fluids
    - ↑ oxytocin gtt
    - Identify lacerated areas and control w/ clamps or direct pressure

- -

ECLAMPSIA (Sz)/ PRE-ECLAMPSIA (PIH)

Acute HTN after the 24th week or an ↑ in SBP of 30 mmHg or an ↑ in DBP of 15 mmHg or more from the baseline during the course of pregnancy. Usually seen w/ primip, teenage primip or primip > 35 yo.

S/S:
- Triad of sx:
    - HTN
    - Proteinuria (> 300 mg/24 hr or > 1+ on urine dipstick)
    - Edema

- HA, N/V, ankle clonus/hyperreflexia, RUQ pain due to subcapsular hepatic hemorrhage which may lead to rupture of the liver capsule
- **Dyspnea, tachypnea, crackles, wheeze, cough, tachycardia = impending eclampsia**
  *Sz due to cerebral edema

- HELLP: **h**emolysis, **el**evated liver enzymes, **l**ow **p**latelet is a form of severe pre-eclampsia

*If pre-eclampsia before the 20th week, think molar pregnancy!

MILD PRE-ECLAMPSIA
- BP 130/80 to 160/110 w/ edema and proteinuria

SEVERE PRE-ECLAMPSIA
- Mild pre-eclampsia + one of the following:
  a. BP > 160/110
  b. Proteinuria > 5 g/24 hr (2+ to 3+ on urine dipstick) or oliguria < 500 ml/24 hr
  c. Neurological Sx: Falls, ↓ LOC, ataxia, scotoma. Sx 2° to vasoconstrictive cerebral ischemia which leads to multifocal petechial hemorrhages @ the gray-white matter junction. (con't)

235

Eclampsia/Pre-Eclampsia (con't)

        d.   RUQ pain: $2°$ stretching of the
               liver capsule due to
               hemorrhage or microinfarctions
               of the liver

Tx:

- Prevent sz: Mg^{++} bolus of 4 – 6 g and a
              gtt @ 2 g/hr @ concentrated
              doses to restrict fluids
  *Monitor for respiratory arrest if the
  patient is taking Ca^{++} channel blockers
  and is receiving Mg^{++}
  *Monitor DTR's

- HTN: hydralazine 5 mg IV then
          5 – 10 mg IV q 20 min depending
          on the BP response
          *GOAL: DBP = 90 – 100 mmHg
  *Tx if BP 160/110 – 120 due to risk of
  CVA, hepatic hemorrhage, placental
  abruption
  *May use labetalol, nitroglycerin,
  nifedipine or nitroprusside instead
  *Hydralazine is contraindicated if the
  patient is tachycardic or if the patient has
  SLE

- Sz: Mg^{++} bolus 4 – 6 g over 15 – 30 min
      or phenytoin 15 – 25 mg/kg @
      25 mg/min
      *May use diazepam to break sz

- Pulmonary Edema: furosemide 20 – 40
                    mg IV and morphine
                    2 – 5 mg IV

- Monitor for DIC
  1. Hgb may be ↑ due to
     hemoconcentration from 3rd spacing
     *Normal Hgb in pregnancy is 9 – 10
     g/dl due to ↑ intravascular volume
  2. Thrombocytopenia is due to TXA_2
     which leads to platelet aggregation
  3. ↑ LFT's
     *↑ ALP is wnl in pregnancy due to
     placental secretion of the enzyme
  4. Uric acid and BUN ↑ due to
     glomerular damage
     *Uric acid is wnl < 6 mg/dl in
     pregnancy due to ↑ GFR
     *Uric acid in non-pregnancy is
     10 – 12 mg/dl
  5. ↓ fibrinogen
  6. ↑ fibrin split products

- -

EFFACEMENT
- Thickness of the cervix expressed as a percent
- Expressed from 0% (thick) to 100% (thin or complete) measured from the fetal head to the external os
- Average cervix is 4 cm thick from the internal os to the external os

```
  0% effaced  =  4 cm thick
 25% effaced  =  3 cm thick
 50% effaced  =  2 cm thick
 75% effaced  =  1 cm thick
100% effaced  =  0 cm thick
```

- - - - - - - - - - - - - - - - - - - -

FETAL HEART MONITORING
1. Determine uterine activity – frequency, duration, intensity
   *Adequate labor is 210 – 250 Montevideo units
   *Montevideo Unit: Sum of the mmHg peaks of each contraction in a 10 min period

2. Fetal Heart Rate
   *FHR should be between 120 – 160 beats per min

*Many term and post term fetuses have a stable baseline between 100 – 120 beats per min. This is wnl if accelerations and adequate variability are present.

*Look at the following 3 areas when determining FHR

A. Baseline – normal, tachycardia, bradycardia
B. Baseline variability – short term, long term
C. Periodic events – accelerations, decelerations, other abnormalities i.e. sinusoidal, fetal hypoxia progression

VARIABILITY:

- Short term (beat-to-beat): ≥ 5 beats above and below baseline. If present means that the baby is in good condition w/ intact cerebral cortex and nervous system.

- Long term: Δ of ≥ 6 beats per min lasting 10 – 20 sec = Δ in long term variability

(con't)

Fetal Heart Monitoring – Variability (con't)
Decreased:
- Medications: narcotics, magnesium, sedatives
- Hypoxia
- Prematurity
- Fetal Sleep
- Tachycardia
- Congenital Anomalies

Increased:
- Fetal Movement
- Early Hypoxia
- Idiopathic

*↓ variability = depressed baby
*At 32 – 34 weeks expect tachycardia and absent beat-to-beat variability

** THIS IS NOT OK @ 35 WEEKS! **

ACCELERATION
- Associated w/ fetal movement
  *Hypoxic/acidotic fetus CAN NOT ↑ HR

BRADYCARDIA: FHR < 120
Moderate: FHR 100 – 120
  *Usually tolerated well by the fetus

Severe: FHR < 100
  *Results in decompensation

240

Causes: FETAL HYPOXIA, severe cord
compression, hypertonic/tetanic
contraction, maternal hypovolemia,
fetal heart block, drugs, severe fetal
blood loss (ruptured vasa previa),
terminal event, idiopathic

*Many term and post term fetuses may have
stable baseline between 100 – 120 beats per
min. This is alright if accelerations and
adequate variability present.
*If rapid drop in HR during pushing @
second stage, delivery will soon follow

TACHYCARDIA: FHR > 160

Causes: Prematurity, maternal fever, smoking,
chorioamnionitis, fetal cardiac
conduction defect, drugs, idiopathic,
anemia, hypovolemia, hypotension

EARLY DECELERATION
- Head compression causing vagal
  stimulation
- Frequently occurs in active labor when
  cervix is dilated to 4 – 7 cm
- Usually not > 20 beats per min
- Benign – no tx needed

(con't)

Fetal Heart Monitoring (con't)
VARIABLE DECELERATION
- Due to transient cord compression
- V or W shaped waveform

Rule of 60's
1. A drop of > 60 beats per min from baseline
2. A drop to below 60 beats per min
3. Deceleration lasting > 60 sec

*Any one is a sign of a severe deceleration

LATE DECELERATION
*Usually very unassuming but most deadly

*To help detect subtle decelerations, turn the monitor strip 90° and look at it vertically
*Usually a late deceleration is no > 20 beats per min
*Late decelerations indicate uteroplacental insufficiency

Causes: Fetal hypoxia, chronic uteroplacental insufficiency, maternal vena caval compression, maternal hypotension, PIH, DM, CV dz, renal dz, placental abruption/previa, uterine hypertonus

BABY NEEDS TO BE DELIVERED

*Late deceleration w/ no variability is an ominous sign

SINUSOIDAL: looks like a sine wave

Causes: Fetal hypovolemia, anemia, erythroblastosis fetalis, abruption

MANAGEMENT OF DECELERATIONS:
1. Identify cause
   *If early deceleration, observe patient
2. If late deceleration, administer O_2, ↑ fluids, place patient in left lateral decubitus position
3. If variable deceleration, amnioinfusion of 500 ml bolus followed by 200 ml/hr
4. Tocolysis
5. Ascertain anticipated time of delivery to determine if baby can be born vaginally or if the patient will need to go for a c-section sooner

*DELIVERY IS THE ONLY CURE

- - - - - - - - - - - - - - - - - - - -

FUNDAL HEIGHT DURING PREGNANCY

8 weeks: @ pubic symphysis

12 weeks: Uterus becomes an abdominal organ

15 weeks: Midway between the pubic symphysis and the umbilicus

20 weeks: @ the umbilicus

20 – 36 weeks: Distance in cm from the symphysis to the fundus = weeks of gestation

----

GROUP B STREPTOCOCCUS (GBS) PROPHYLAXIS

Mothers w/ GBS (+) cultures in 3rd Trimester

Risks:

1. Gestation < 37 weeks
2. PROM > 24 hr
3. Maternal intrapartum fever

Tx:

- Ampicillin 2 g IV followed by 1 g q 4 hr until delivery

OR

- 5 million units PCN-G IV followed by 2.5 million units q 4 hr until delivery

*Administer GBS prophylaxis to the neonate
- If sx of infection present, i.e. tachypnea, temperature regulation difficulties, etc.
- If the neonate is premature
- An asymptomatic newborn w/ twin (+) for GBS

- -

β-HCG LEVELS

Gestational Age	HCG Levels (mIU/ml)
7 – 10 days	> 3
30 days	100 – 5000
10 weeks	50,000 – 140,000
> 16 weeks	10,000 – 50,000

*When HCG level is 2000, vaginal ultrasound should be able to detect a gestational sac
*When HCG level is 6000, abdominal ultrasound should be able to detect a gestational sac

- -

INCOMPETENT CERVIX
Seen midtrimester between 18 to 24 weeks

S/S: Hourglassing of membranes

Tx:
- Trendelenberg position
- Tocolytic

*Nothing can be done if the membranes rupture
*Generally the fetus must be @ least 24 weeks for viability

- -

OBSTETRICS TRANSFER SHEET

1. Maternal Hx:
   - Age of patient
   - Gravida
   - Para: Term, Preterm, Abortions, Living
   - Weeks gestation
   - FDLMP
   - Estimated Date of Confinement (Delivery)
   - Onset of contractions
   - Frequency of contractions
   - Cervical dilation
   - Last checked, by whom

*If in **active labor** or history of incompetent cervix or precipitous delivery, vaginal exam should have been done within **30 min** prior to transport
*If < **34 weeks** gestation and > **4 cm** dilated, contact **receiving** physician or medical control for consultation prior to transport

2. ROM: Y or N
   - If yes, most recent cervical dilation assessment after rupture. Note cm, time and performed by whom
   - If yes, is meconium staining present?

3. Evidence of vaginal bleeding: Y or N

(con't)

Obstetrics Transfer Sheet (con't)

4. FHR and time last obtained
   *If multiple pregnancy obtain for each fetus

5. Blood type

6. Perinatal Hx

7. MgSO$_4$ Infusing: Y or N
   - If yes, DTR's and time for the last two sets

8. Referring and receiving physician name and phone number

- -

PLACENTA PREVIA

Painless bright red vaginal bleeding in the 3rd trimester (mean age of dx is 32 wks) due to abnormal implantation of the placenta in the lower uterine segment

- ***Vaginal exam contraindicated!***
- Monitor for DIC w/ wall clot test:
  Place 5 ml of blood in a red top tube, place upright. If there is no clot formation within in 6 – 12 min or if clot lysis occurs within 30 min an abnormality in clotting may be present.
  *Can be used if lab is not available

*If not profusely bleeding, it is safe to transfer
*1 soaked pad = 20 – 30 ml of blood

Tx:
- 2 large bore IV's
- Type and cross
- Prepare for c-section if massive hemorrhage
- Continuous fetal monitoring

- -

PREMATURE RUPTURE OF MEMBRANES (PROM)

ROM prior to the onset of labor @ any stage of gestation, usually 1 – 2 hr before the onset of contractions

*Preterm ROM (PPROM): ROM prior to 37 weeks gestation w/ or w/o contractions

Tx:
- If contracting, check dilation
  *Membranes normally rupture when dilated to 4 – 5 cm, definite rupture by 6 – 8 cm
- Check FHR
- Start IV
- If labor starts, administer a tocolytic
- Check for cord prolapse
  - If present, transport in Trendelenberg position or knee-chest position

*∅ replace the cord, may cause severe cord compression

- -

PRETERM LABOR

*Always think of infectious etiology for PTL
*Term: > 37 wks
 Preterm: 20 – 37 wks
 Ab: < 20 wks

False Labor: Typically irregular contractions
              > 5 min apart w/ no cervical Δ's

True Labor: Typically regular contractions
             5 min apart or less w/ cervical Δ's

Tx:
-   IV hydration
-   Tocolytic – Mg^{++}, terbutaline, ritodrine
    *∅ mix tocolytics
-   Nalbuphine (Nubain) up to 10 mg IV over
    3 – 5 min

**Will the patient deliver enroute?
-   If primipara, alright to transport
-   **Multiparous patient dilated 4 – 5 cm is
    considered to be an imminent delivery**
- -

STAGES OF LABOR
First Stage
- Latent: Onset of labor to 4 cm dilation
    - Nulliparous: Average 8 hr
                *No > 20 hr
    - Parous: Average 5 hr
                *No > 14 hr

- Active: 4 cm dilation to complete dilation
    - Nulliparous: Average 5 hr
                *No > 12 hr
        *Should progress @ least 1 cm/hr
    - Parous: Average 2 hr
                *No > 5 hr
        *Should progress @ least 2 cm/hr

Second Stage
- Complete dilation to delivery of the infant
    *Patient feels like they want to push or
    move their bowels
    *Second stage should not last > 3 hr
    - Nulliparous: Average 1 – 2 hr
    - Parous: Average 30 min

Third Stage
- Delivery of the infant to delivery of the
  placenta and membranes
- Usually no > 30 min
- Average is 10 min or less

*Brandt-Andrews Maneuver:
-    Stimulation of the fundus to
     cause contractions, followed by
     suprapubic pressure directed
     down toward the sacrum then
     upward toward the fundus
     *Used to aid separation of the
     placenta from the uterus

*If > 30 min pass before the placenta is
delivered, be concerned about a retained
placenta
*Place the patient on an oxytocin gtt after
delivery of the placenta is complete

Fourth Stage
-    Delivery of the placenta to 1 hr
     post-partum
-    Monitor for excessive vaginal bleeding
-    90% of cases of post-partum hemorrhage
     are from uterine atony
     -    Tx uterine atony
          -    Uterine massage
          -    Oxytocin gtt

- -

STATION

- Level of the presenting part in relationship to the ischial spines
- Expressed as "minus" above the ischial spines, "0" @ the level of the ischial spines (engaged) and "plus" when below the ischial spines
- -3, -2, -1, 0 (@ ischial spines – engaged), +1, +2, +3 (crowning)

Ballottment: Pushing on the fetal head and feeling it bounce back against your fingers. A fetal head that can be ballotted is unengaged or floating.

- - - - - - - - - - - - - - - - - - - -

BRONCHIOLITIS

Inflammatory destruction of the small airways
w/ mucous plugging and intraluminal debris
- Children < 2 yo (< 6 mo greatest
  incidence)
- October to May presentation
- Respiratory Syncytial Virus (RSV)
  accounts for 75 – 90% of cases
  *Parainfluenza or influenza may be
  causative
  *Adenovirus may be causative and lead
  to Bronchiolitis Obliterans Organizing
  Pneumonia (BOOP)

Dx:
- Preceding URI symptoms
- Rapid respirations
- Retractions
- Wheezing
- CXR: Hyperinflation w/ small areas
  of atelectasis or patchy
  infiltrates

Tx:
- Humidified O_2 @ 28 – 40%
  FiO_2
- Airway intervention prn*
- Fluids: rehydration and
  maintenance
- Albuterol (0.03 ml) 0.15
  mg/kg/dose in 2 ml NS
  aerosolized prn

(con't)

255

Bronchiolitis (con't)

- Consider racemic epinephrine 0.05 – 0.1 ml/kg of 2.25% sol'n if albuterol fails
- Ribavirin (Virazole)
    - 6 gm aerosolized over 18 – 20 hr qd × 3 – 5 d

    OR

    - 2 gm aerosolized over 2 hrs q 8 hr × 3 – 5 d

    *Use only if confirmed RSV, patient NOT improving, or for high risk patients i.e. BPD, congenital heart disease

*Consider CPAP or intubation if
- ↑ RR
- ↑ HR
- ↑ $PaCO_2$
- ↓ PaO_2
- ↓ LOC

*ECMO has been shown to be effective treatment if the patient fails these measures
*Glucocorticoids, ipratropium and theophylline are NOT beneficial

- -

CROUP
(LaryngoTracheoBronchitis)

Acute viral illness which leads to a gradually worsening, barky cough especially at night

- Children 6 mo – 3 yrs
- Fall through Winter presentation
- Parainfluenza most likely causative agent
  *RSV and influenza may also be causative

Dx:

- Preceding URI
- Stridor
- Barky cough
- Retractions
- Tachypnea
- Hoarseness
- CXR: Steeple Sign

Tx:

- Humidified O_2 – Cool Mist
- Racemic epinephrine 0.05 – 0.1 ml/kg aerosolized
- Dexamethasone 0.6 mg/kg IV/IM/PO q 6 – 12 hr × 1 – 4 doses
- Hydration IV or PO
- Antipyretics
- Intubation for respiratory failure

*Antibiotics are only needed in a bacterial infection is present along w/ croup

- -

DIABETIC KETOACIDOSIS – PEDS

Dx:
- Glucose > 300 mg/dl
- Metabolic acidosis per ABG
  - PH < 7.30
  - HCO_3 < 15 mEq/L
- Ketonemia
- Ketonuria

*Obtain electrolytes, BUN, Cr, glucose, CBC, ABG, UA, amylase, lipase, serum osmolality
*If ketone/fruity breath expect pH to be < 7.12

Tx: Child:
- Assume 5 – 10% dehydration
- Give 10 – 20 ml/kg NS or LR over 1 hr, then start 0.45 NS as follows:
  - Replace the remaining deficit **plus** the maintenance requirements over 36 – 48 hrs
- Start regular insulin gtt at 0.1 U/kg/hr if hemodynamically stable
- Obtain serum glucose q 1 hr, CBG q 2 hr until pH > 7.35
  *This therapy should lower serum glucose by 80 – 100 mg/dl/hr
  - If glucose falls faster, continue insulin gtt @ 0.1 U/kg/hr and add D_5W to IV fluid after there are no ketones in the urine and serum
- Start feeding when HCO_3 > 16

*When serum glucose < 300 mg/dl, add D_5W and continue insulin gtt @ 0.1 U/kg/hr

*When serum glucose < 250 mg/dl and the patient is NOT spilling ketones in urine, discontinue insulin gtt 1 – 2 hr after administration of SQ insulin and administer SQ insulin as follows:
  - For the first 24 hrs give regular insulin 0.1 – 0.25 U/kg SQ q 6 – 8 hr
  - Obtain serum glucose q 6 hr and PRN

*$\emptyset \downarrow$ insulin dose based on plasma glucose. May lead to exacerbation of ketosis and acidosis. Rather, $\uparrow$ the concentration of dextrose so that the insulin gtt can be maintained @ 0.1U/kg/hr until acidosis is resolved.

*$NaHCO_3$ is generally not indicated since rehydration and insulin administration will correct the acidosis

*There is total body depletion of K^+ w/ DKA. Begin w/ 20 – 40 mEq/L of K^+ if the patient is hypokalemic, normokalemic and has good UO.
*Check serum K^+ q 2 hrs

(con't)

Diabetic Ketoacidosis – Peds (con't)
*HPO_4, which is depleted in DKA, will drop w/ insulin therapy. PO_4 improves release of O_2 to tissues. Therefore, replace PRN and consider replacing K^+ as ½ KCl and ½ KPO_4 for the first 8 hr, then all as KCl after 8 hr.
*Excessive PO_4 may induce hypocalcemic tetany

IV FLUID ADMINISTRATION
- If FSBS > 300, use 0.45 NS w/ 2 mEq KCl/100 ml
- If FSBS > 150 but < 300, use $D_5$0.45NS w/ 2 mEq KCl/100 ml
- If FSBS < 150 use D_{10}0.45NS w/ 2 mEq KCl/100 ml

- - - - - - - - - - - - - - - - - - - -

ELECTROLYTE DISTURBANCES
Hypocalcemia: Serum Ca^{++} < 8.5 mg/dl or ionized Ca^{++} < 4.40 mg/dl
Circumoral paresthesias, paresthesias of the digits, sz, Chovstek's sign, Trousseau's sign

Causes: Hypoparathyroidism, pseudohypoparathyroidism, vitamin D deficiency, renal failure, magnesium deficiency, multiple blood transfusions

*If the patient has hypoalbuminemia, adjust the Ca^{++} level as follows:

Adjusted Ca^{++} =
Serum Ca^{++} + 0.8 × (4 − albumin)

Tx: Child: Ca^{++} gluconate:
- 200 − 500 mg/kg/d IV/PO ÷ q 6 hr

Infant: Ca^{++} gluconate:
- 200 − 500 mg/kg/d IV ÷ q 6 hr
- 400 − 800 mg/kg/d PO ÷ q 6 hr

Neonate: Ca^{++} gluconate:
- 200 − 800 mg/kg/d IV ÷ q 6 hr

Hypercalcemia: Serum Ca^{++} > 10.5 mg/dl or ionized Ca^{++} < 5.4 mg/dl
Anorexia, N/V, constipation, muscle weakness, polyuria, polydipsia, neurotic behavior, dysrhythmias

Causes: Hyperparathyroidism, ectopic PTH-producing tumors, vitamin D excess, malignancy, immobilization

(con't)

261

Electrolyte Dist – Hypercalcemia (con't)
Tx: Child:

- IV NS @ 200 – 250 ml/kg/d
- Furosemide 1 mg/kg q 6 hr
- Hydrocortisone 1 mg/kg q 6 hr
  *↓ intestinal absorption of Ca^{++}
- Calcitonin 10 U/kg IV q 4 hr
- Etrodinate if unresponsive to above measures

Hypokalemia: Serum K^+ < 3.5 mEq/L
Anorexia, N/V, fatigue, muscle weakness, ↓ bowel motility, dysrhythmias, paresthesias, flat T-waves on ECG, MAT

Causes: Renovascular dz, excess renin, excess mineralocorticoid, Cushing's syndrome, renal tubular acidosis, antibiotics, diuretics, cystic fibrosis, skin losses, GI losses, alkalosis, excessive insulin, leukemia

Tx: Child: 1 – 2 mEq KCl/kg IV slowly @
0.5 – 1.0 mEq/kg/hr
MAX: 20 mEq/hr

Hyperkalemia: Serum K^+ > 5.8 mEq/L
Dysrhythmias, bradycardia, muscle weakness, flaccid paralysis, tall tented T-waves on ECG

Causes: Cell breakdown, congenital adrenal hypoplasia, renal failure, hemolysis, hypoaldosteronism, aldosterone insensitivity, low insulin, K^+-sparing diuretics, leukocytosis, metabolic acidosis, thrombocytosis

Tx: Child:

- 0.2 – 0.5 ml/kg (minimum 10 ml) 10% Ca gluconate IV over 2 – 5 min
  *Effective for up to 1 hr
  *Temporarily stabilizes cardiac cell membrane
- $D_5$0.45 NaCl w/ 40 mEq/L $NaHCO_3$ infused at 20 ml/kg/hr × 1 – 2 hr
  *↓ K^+ in ECF via volume expansion of ECF
- 1 – 3 mEq/kg $NaHCO_3$ over 3 – 5 min
  *Lasts several hours
  *↓ ECF K^+

(con't)

263

Electrolyte Dist – Hyperkalemia (con't)

- 0.5 – 1.0 g/kg glucose w/ 0.3 U regular insulin/g glucose over 1 – 2 hr
  *↓ ECF K^+
- Albuterol aerosols
  *↓ ECF K^+
- 1 mg/kg furosemide over 1 – 2 min
  *Removes K^+ from body
- Kayexalate 1 – 2 g/kg w/ 3 ml sorbitol/g resin PO ÷ q 6 hr
  OR
- Kayexalate 1 – 2 g/kg w/ 5 ml sorbitol/g resin PR over 4 – 6 hr
- Emergent dialysis PRN

Hypomagnesemia: Serum Mg^{++} < 1.5 mEq/L Dysrhythmias, neuromuscular irritability, disorientation

Causes: Furosemide, aminoglycosides, digitalis, diarrhea, alcohol abuse, DM, acute MI

Tx: Child: 25 – 50 mg/kg q 4 – 6 hr × 3 – 4 doses

Hypermagnesemia: Serum Mg^{++} > 2.5 mEq/L
Hypotension, flushing,
drowsiness, ↓ DTR's,
respiratory depression,
coma, cardiac arrest

Causes: Impaired renal function

Tx: Child:
- Hemodialysis
- Ca^{++} gluconate: dosing for age
- If patient can tolerate fluids,
  aggressive fluid administration
  w/ furosemide may be effective

Hyponatremia: Serum Na$^+$ < 135 mEq/L
Anorexia, N/V, confusion,
lethargy, muscle cramps,
muscular twitching, sz,
papilledema

Causes: GI loss, third spacing, skin loss,
nephrotic syndrome, CHF, SIADH,
factitious

(desired Na$^+$ − actual Na$^+$) × 0.6 × kg wt =
mEq Na$^+$ to replace

*In children use D$_5$0.45NaCl

(con't)

Electrolyte Dist – Hyponatremia (con't)
*Hyperglycemia:
- $Na^+ \downarrow$ by 1.6 mEq/L for q 100 mg/dl $\uparrow$ in glucose

*Hyperproteinemia:
- $Na^+ \downarrow$ by $0.25 \times [protein (g/dl) - 8]$

*Hyperlipidemia:
- $Na^+ \downarrow 0.002 \times lipid (mg/dl)$

*For hyponatremia **not** caused by dehydration, fluid restriction is indicated until the serum sodium normalizes

Hypernatremia: Serum $Na^+ > 145$ mEq/L
Thirst, $\uparrow$ temperature, edematous dry tongue, tenacious sputum, hallucinations, lethargy, irritability, focal or grand mal sz, hyperreflexia

Causes: $\downarrow$ free H_2O intake, GI loss, skin loss, diuretics, nephropathy, diabetes insipidus, excess Na^+ administration, mineralocorticoid excess

$$H_2O \text{ deficit} = \frac{\text{serum } Na^+ - 140}{140} \times 0.6 \times \text{kg wt}$$

Tx:
- If hypovolemic replace volume first w/ NS or LR until BP and tissue perfusion are adequate
- Next, use $D_5 0.33$ NaCl or $D_5 0.2$ NaCl
- Add Ca^{++} as needed

*NOTE: $\emptyset$ correct faster than 10 – 15 mEq/L/d (0.5 mEq/L/hr) due to risk of cerebral edema, sz, pulmonary edema and death

*Each liter of H_2O deficit raises the serum Na^+ by 3 – 5 mEq/L
*Add 20 – 40 mEq KCl/L which aids water entry into the cells
*Replace total fluid deficit over 48 – 72 hrs

Hypophosphatemia: Serum PO_4 < 3.0 mg/dl Muscle weakness, pain and tenderness, mental status Δ's, respiratory failure, paresthesias, cardiomyopathy

Causes: Phosphate binding antacids, renal tubular phosphate reabsorption defects, movement of PO_4 into cells

(con't)

Electrolyte Dist – Hypophosphatemia (con't)

Tx: Child: 0.15 – 0.33 mmol/kg IV over 6 hrs
              OR
              15 – 45 mg/kg/d po ÷ BID
              *Infuse at ≤ 0.1 mmol/kg/hr
              MAX: 0.2 mmol/kg/hr
              *Infusion may cause hypotension

Hyperphosphatemia: Serum PO_4 > 4.0
                        mg/dl

Short term: Circumoral paresthesias,
             paresthesias of the digits, sx of
             tetany

Long term: Precipitation of $CaPO_4$ in
            non-osseous sites

Causes: Renal insufficiency, widespread cell
         necrosis, DKA, hypoparathyroidism,
         pseudohypoparathyroidism

Tx: Dietary restriction, phosphate binders i.e.
     aluminum containing antacids

- -

EPIGLOTTITIS

Acute, life-threatening pediatric emergency caused by inflammation of the epiglottis which may lead to airway obstruction

- Can occur at any age, but peak incidence is 2 – 5 yo
- Any season
- Causative agent is Haemophilus influenzae

Dx:

- Abrupt onset
- Toxic appearing
- High fever
- Sore throat
- Stridor
- Dysphagia
- Drooling
- Whispering voice

Tx:

- DO NOT upset the child
- Immediate intubation in a controlled setting
- Allow patient to breath on own w/ humidified O_2 and CPAP of 4 – 6 mmHg

(con't)

Epiglottitis – Tx (con't)

- Cefuroxime (Zinacef)
  100 – 150 mg/kg/d ÷ q 6 – 8 hr
  IV

  OR

  Cefotaxime (Claforan)
  50 – 150 mg/kg/d ÷ q 6 – 8 hr
  IV

  OR

  Ceftriaxone (Rocephin)
  50 – 75 mg/kg/d ÷ q 12 hr IV
  *Switch to oral after extubation
   so that the patient receives a
   full 10 day course

*Extubate after 36 – 48 hrs if clinically
 indicated

– – – – – – – – – – – – – – – – – – – –

EXTRACORPOREAL MEMBRANE OXYGENATION – THE BASICS

Use: Extracorporeal oxygenation of the blood and organ perfusion for neonates w/ severe cardiopulmonary failure

Indications: Meconium aspiration syndrome, respiratory distress syndrome, sepsis, persistent pulmonary HTN of the newborn

Pediatric/Adult ECMO Eligibility

- Ventilator support > 7 d
- Ventilator settings
    - PIP > 35 cm H_2O
    - PEEP > 10 cm H_2O
    - Mean airway pressure > 18 cm H_2O
- Oxygenation Index (OI) > 40
- PaO_2/FiO_2 < 150
- ≥ 34 weeks gestation
- ≥ 2.5 kg
- Failure of other therapies
    - Inverse I/E ratio ventilation
    - Nitric oxide inhalation
    - High frequency ventilation
    - Surfactant
    - Permissive hypercapnia
    - Liquid ventilation

(con't)

ECMO (con't)
Selection Criteria:

- Alveolar-arterial oxygenation difference
  ($AaDO_2$) > 610 for 8 hr or > 605 for 4 hr if
  PIP > 38 cm H_2O
  *Predicts a mortality > 80%
  *$AaDO_2 = (760 - 47) \times F_iO_2 - 1.2(PaCO_2)$

- Oxygenation Index (OI) > 40
  *Predicts a mortality > 90%
- OI 25 – 40
  *Predicts a mortality of 50 – 80%

- PaO_2 < 40 mmHg × 2 hr and/or pH
  < 7.15 × 2 hr
- PaO_2 < 55 mmHg and pH < 7.40 × 3 hr

- Any 4 of the following:
  - Pneumothorax
  - Pneumomediastinum
  - Pneumoperitoneum
  - Pulmonary interstitial emphysema
  - Persistent air leak > 24 hr
  - Mean airway pressure > 15 cm H_2O
  - Subcutaneous emphysema

Usual duration of ECMO:
48 – 72 hr: RDS
72 + 24 hr: Sepsis
72 + 24 + 24 hr: Diaphragmatic hernia

ECMO Flow Rates:
- Start at 50 ml/kg/min
- ↑ by 50 – 100 ml/kg/min until usual flow is reached

  *Flow is ↑ in sepsis
- Usual flow is as follows:
  - Neonate: 100 – 120 ml/kg/min × 0.8
  - Child: 90 ml/kg/min × 0.8
  - Adult: 70 ml/kg/min × 0.8

    *80% is the maximum amount of the patient's CO that should be pulled off to go through the pump. If more CO is pulled off, it may lead to pulmonary alkalosis or direct pulmonary capillary damage

- To ↑ the PaO_2:
  - ↑ flow
  - Diurese the fluid overloaded patient

    *↑ ventilator FiO_2 or ↑ sweep will not ↑ PaO_2

Lab Goals:
- Hct ≥ 35
- PTT < 150
- Platelet count 80,000 – 100,000
- Normal fibrinogen level of 200 – 400
- Normal electrolytes
- SaO_2 ≥ 95

*Correct the above as needed with the appropriate therapies

ECMO (con't)
Weaning from ECMO:

- $\downarrow$ flow by 10 – 20 ml/min if PaO_2 > 60 torr and venous saturation > 65%
- When flow is 60 – 70 ml/kg/min
  - $\uparrow$ ventilator settings to a PIP 20 – 30 cm H_2O
  - Rate 20 – 30
  - FiO_2 0.3 – 0.4
  - PEEP 5 cm H_2O
- Wean until flow is 50 – 100 ml/min and PaO_2 and venous saturations > 65%
- Clamp the cannulas and observe the patient
- If the patient remains stable, i.e. adequate oxygenation and ventilation, and hemodynamically stable, the patient can be decannulated

Complications: Bleeding/major hemorrhage, intracranial hemorrhage (13% neonates, 5% pediatric), infection, neurologic damage, ischemia

- -

HIGH-FREQUENCY OSCILLATION VENTILATION

Indications:

- Airleaks
  - Pulmonary interstitial emphysema
  - Bronchopulmonary fistula
  - Pneumothorax

  *GOAL: Lung protection by using mean airway pressure (P_{aw}) $\leq$ conventional mechanical ventilation (CMV)

- Respiratory Failure
  - RDS
  - Pneumonia
  - Meconium aspiration
  - Primary pulmonary HTN
  - Tracheoesophageal fistula
  - Pulmonary hemorrhage

- Lung Hypoplasia Syndromes
  - Congenital diaphragmatic hernia
  - Hydrops fetalis
  - Potters variant

Inclusion Criteria:

- Oxygenation Index (OI) > 13 in two ABG's within a 6 hr period
  *Assure adequate BP
  *If pH < 7.28 consider using THAM

(con't)

HFOV (con't)
Exclusion Criteria:
- Dx of RSV
- ↑ airway resistance
- ↑ ICP
- Wt > 70 kg
- MAP < 55 mmHg

Initial Settings
- Start w/ FiO_2 1.0

- Start w/ a P_{aw} 4 – 8 cmH_2O above the P_{aw} on CMV
  *↑ P_{aw} in 1 – 2 cmH_2O increments until optimal lung volume:
    - ↑ SaO_2 will be seen allowing a ↓ in F_iO_2 < 0.6
    - CXR shows the diaphragms at T9

- Set Bias Flow Rate:
    - Premature: 10 – 15 lpm
    - Near-term: 10 – 20 lpm
    - Small child: 15 – 25 lpm
    - Large child: 20 – 30 lpm
    *MAX: 40 lpm

  *Monitor window = P_{aw} + Bias flow
  *P_{aw} limit = P_{aw} + 10 cmH_2O
  *Adjust flow to obtain desired P_{aw}

- Set frequency
  - < 1000 g: 15 Hz
  - 1000 – 2000 g: 12 Hz
  - 2 – 12 kg: 10 Hz
  - 13 – 20 kg: 8 Hz
  - 21 – 30 kg: 7 Hz
  - 31 – 60 kg: 6 Hz
  - *1 Hz = 60 breaths

- Set ΔP (Amplitude)
  - Neonate: 2.0
  - Pediatric: 4.0
    * NOT uncommon for the $PaCO_2$ to initially rise for up to 2 hr before decreasing
    - $\uparrow$ the amplitude in 5 cm increments until the max ΔP is reached, then $\downarrow$ frequency
    - If no (+) effect is achieved, $\downarrow$ the frequency by 1 Hz
    - Maintain the I-time at 33% until the amplitude has been $\uparrow$ to the maximum and then $\downarrow$ the frequency to 3 Hz if needed

- Assess Chest Wiggle Factor (CWF)
  - Neonates: CW should not be below the umbilical area
  - Children: CW should not be below the groin area

(con't)

HFOV – Initial Settings (con't)
- Set I-time (% Inspiratory Time):
  - 33% preterm
  - 33 – 50% pediatric

Helpful Hints:
- Initiate HFOV when $PaCO_2$ reaches 60 – 70 mmHg
- Confirm adequate ventilation w/ CXR – should see the diaphragms at T9
- ALL patients > 10 kg should receive neuromuscular blockade and sedation
- IO < 42 @ 24 hrs of HFOV is a good indicator of a (+) response
- Maintain wnl MAP (no < 60 mmHg)
- ↑ CVP to 15 – 20 mmHg by giving volume
- Maintain PCWP ≥ 15 mmHg
  *If PCWP is unavailable and the CVP is 15 – 20 mmHg with a MAP < 60 mmHg, start a dobutamine gtt at 5 – 20 µg/kg/min
- Oxygenation is affected by:
  - P_{aw}
  - ΔP – when inflation is inadequate
  - Frequency (Hz) – to a lesser degree
- Ventilation is affected by:
  - ΔP
  - Frequency – CO_2 follows the same direction as the frequency
  - I-time

HFOV Management

- $FiO_2 > 0.6$
    - $PaCO_2 \uparrow$ w/
        - $PaO_2 \uparrow$: $\uparrow \Delta P, \downarrow FiO_2$
        - PaO_2 wnl: $\uparrow \Delta P$
        - $PaO_2 \downarrow$: $\uparrow P_{aw}, \uparrow \Delta P, \uparrow FiO_2$

- $FiO_2 > 0.6$
    - $PaCO_2$ wnl w/
        - $PaO_2 \uparrow$: $\downarrow FiO_2$
        - PaO_2 wnl: No change needed
        - $PaO_2 \downarrow$: $\uparrow P_{aw}, \uparrow FiO_2$

- $FiO_2 > 0.6$
    - $PaCO_2 \downarrow$ w/
        - $PaO_2 \uparrow$: $\downarrow FiO_2, \downarrow \Delta P$
        - PaO_2 wnl: $\downarrow \Delta P$
        - $PaO_2 \downarrow$: $\uparrow P_{aw}, \uparrow FiO_2, \downarrow \Delta P$

- $FiO_2 < 0.6$
    - $PaCO_2 \uparrow$ w/:
        - $PaO_2 \uparrow$: $\uparrow \Delta P, \downarrow P_{aw}$
        - PaO_2 wnl: $\uparrow \Delta P$
        - $PaO_2 \downarrow$: $\uparrow FiO_2, \uparrow \Delta P$

- $FiO_2 < 0.6$
    - $PaCO_2$ wnl w/:
        - $PaO_2 \uparrow$: $\downarrow P_{aw}, \downarrow FiO_2$
        - PaO_2 wnl: No change needed
        - $PaO_2 \downarrow$: $\uparrow FiO_2$

(con't)

279

HFOV – Management (con't)

- $FiO_2 < 0.6$
    - $PaCO_2 \downarrow$ w/:
        - $PaO_2 \uparrow$: $\downarrow P_{aw}$, $\downarrow \Delta P$
        - PaO_2 wnl: $\downarrow \Delta P$
        - $PaO_2 \downarrow$: $\uparrow FiO_2$, $\downarrow \Delta P$

Failure Criteria:
- Inability to $\downarrow F_iO_2$ by 10% within the first 24 hrs
- Inability to improve or maintain ventilation ($PaCO_2 < 80$ mmHg w/ pH > 7.27)
- Inability to maintain oxygenation – **Contact ECMO center**

Weaning from HFOV:
- $\downarrow F_iO_2$ to < 0.4 to maintain an $SaO_2 > 90\%$
- $\downarrow P_{aw}$ to < 20 cm H_2O in increments of 1 cmH_2O, once $F_iO_2 < 0.6$ and CXR confirms adequate inflation
- $\downarrow \Delta P$ in increments of 5 cmH_2O until $PaCO_2 <$ desired level
- Patient tolerates suctioning w/o $\downarrow SaO_2$
- Once an optimal frequency is found, $\varnothing$ adjust it further

Converting from HFOV to CMV

Convert patient to CMV when:

- $F_iO_2 < 0.4$
- P_{aw} 12 – 20 cmH$_2$O
- $\Delta P < 40$ cmH$_2$O
- Patient has plateaued at specific settings for several days
- Secretions become a problem
- Patient tolerates manual resuscitation

- -

LEVEL OF CONSCIOUSNESS – ALTERED, PEDIATRIC

A

- Alcohol
- Acid/Base and Metabolic Disorders
    - DM, dehydration, hypercapnia, hepatic failure, hypoxia, inborn errors of metabolism
- Arrhythmia/Cardiogenic
    - VF, Stokes-Adams, aortic stenosis

E

- Encephalopathy
    - HTN, Reye's Syndrome, shock
- Endocrinopathy
    - Addison's, congenital adrenal hyperplasia, thyrotoxicity, Cushing's, pheochromocytoma
- Electrolytes

(con't)

LOC – Altered, Pediatric (con't)

I
- Insulin
- Intussusception

O
- Opiates

U
- Uremia
  - CRF, hemolytic uremic syndrome

T
- Trauma
- Thermal
- Tumor

I
- Infection
  - Meningitis, encephalitis, cerebral abscess, sepsis
- Intracerebral Vascular Disorders
  - Arterial/venous thrombosis, intracranial bleed, cerebral embolus

P
- Psychogenic
- Poisoning

S
- Seizure

- - - - - - - - - - - - - - - -

NEONATAL RESUSCITATION OVERVIEW

Initial Steps:

1. Prevent Heat Loss:
   - Place on warmer
   - Dry thoroughly
   - Remove wet towel

2. Open Airway:
   - Position
   - Suction **mouth** first
   - Suction nose

3. Evaluate Infant:
   - Breathing:

     - YES
       - Evaluate HR

     - NO or Gasping
       - PPV w/ 100% O_2 @ 40 – 60 breaths per minute, provide tactile stimulation

*After spontaneous respirations, d/c ventilation and provide initial free-flow O_2 PRN and tactile stimulation

(con't)

Neonatal Resuscitation (con't)

- Intubate if:
    - Prolonged PPV required
    - BVM ineffective
    - Tracheal suctioning required
    - Diaphragmatic hernia

- Heart Rate:
    - > 100: Evaluate color
    - < 100: PPV w/ 100% O_2 for 15 – 30 seconds
    - **If after 15 – 30 seconds**
        - HR > 100: Watch for spontaneous respirations
        - HR 60 – 100
            - HR ↑: Continue PPV
            - HR NOT ↑: PPV
              *If HR < 80, initiate chest compressions for 30 seconds, then reevaluate
              *Meds if HR NOT ↑

- Color:
    - Pink or Acrocyanosis: No tx needed

    - Central Cyanosis: Free flow O_2 if breathing, PPV if not breathing

ETT Size

Weight, g	Gestational Age, wk	Size, mm
Below 1000	Below 28	2.5
1000 – 2000	28 – 34	3.0
2000 – 3000	34 – 38	3.5
Above 3000	Above 38	3.5 – 4.0

Umbilical Venous Catheter:

- < 2 kg use a 3.5 F
- > 2 kg use a 5.0 F

*Use catheters w/ a single end hole and a radiopaque marker

- Emergency Insertion:
    - Insert into the umbilical vein just below the level of the skin
    *A free flow of blood should be present

- Non-Emergency Insertion:
    - Measure from the lateral clavicle (shoulder) to the umbilicus and multiply by 0.6
    *This will place the catheter tip above the diaphragm

Umbilical Arterial Catheter:

Estimated depth of insertion = kg wt + 7 cm

(con't)

285

Neonatal Resuscitation (con't)
Medications

Meds	Conc	Dose/ Route	Note
Epinephrine	1:10,000	0.1 – 0.3 ml/kg IV 1-2 ml/kg/ET	Give rapid IV push
Volume Expanders	Whole blood, 5% albumin, NS, LR	10 ml/kg IV	Give over 5 – 10 min Maintain pH > 7.25
Glucose *see below	D₁₀W	2 – 4 ml/kg IV gtt @ 6 – 8 mg/kg/min	Max rate of infusion: 4 – 15 mg/kg/min
NaHCO₃	4.2 % sol'n (0.5 mEq/ml)	2 mEq/kg IV (4 ml/kg)	Give slowly over @ least 2 min
Naloxone	0.4 mg/ml or 1.0 mg/ml	0.1 mg/kg IV/ET/IM/SQ (0.25 ml/kg) (0.1 ml/kg)	Give rapid IV push
Dopamine	Per formula	5 μg/kg/min May ↑ to 20 μg/kg/min	Infusion pump

Meds	Conc	Dose/ Route	Note
Gentamycin		2.5 mg/kg IV q 12 – 24 hr	Gp B Strep prophylaxis against RDS, sepsis
Ampicillin		< 2 kg: 25 – 50 mg/kg q 12 hr IV ≥ 2 kg: 25 – 50 mg/kg q 8 hr IV	Gp B Strep prophylaxis against RDS, sepsis
Beractant (Survanta)		4 ml/kg via ETT in 4 quarter doses w/ PPV between each dose. MR q 6 hr	MAX: 4 doses Give in downward incline w/ head R and L, and upward incline w/ head R and L
Colfosceril (Exosurf)		5 ml/kg via ETT in 4 quarter doses w/ PPV	2nd dose in 12 hr. Suction within 2 hr only if needed

(con't)

Neonatal Resuscitation (con't)
Rule of 6
n × 6 × kg wt = mg to add to 100 ml of fluid
*1 ml/hr = n μg/kg/min

n = Drug concentration

*n = 0.1 for isoproterenol, epinephrine,
    norepinephrine
*n = 0.3 for prostaglandin
*n = 1 for dopamine, dobutamine,
    nitroprusside
*n = 10 for lidocaine

APGAR Score

Sign	0	1	2
HR/minute	Absent	< 100	> 100
Respirations	Absent	Slow, irreg.	Good, crying
Muscle tone	Limp	Some flexion	Active motion
Reflex irritability (place catheter in nares)	No response	Grimace	Cough or sneeze
Color	Blue or pale	Acrocyanosis	Pink

APGAR Grading

APGAR Score	Classification	pH Range
7 – 10	Normal	≥ 7.20
5 – 6	Mild depression	7.10 – 7.19
3 – 4	Moderate depression	7.00 – 7.09
0 – 2	Severe depression	< 7.00

Blood Gases – Fetal

> 7.25 = wnl
7.20 – 7.24 = preacidotic
< 7.20 = acidotic

Cord Gases – Normal Values

pH: 7.30 – 7.40
pO_2: 15 – 25
pCO_2: 40 – 50
HCO_3: 29 – 39

Neonatal Vital Signs

KG WT	SBP	DBP	HR	RR*	ETT	CT
< 1	40-60	15-35	>100	60-90	2.5	10
1-2	50-60	20-40	>100	60-90	3.0	10-12
2-3	50-70	25-45	>100	60-90	3.5	12
> 3	50-80	30-50	>100	60-90	3.5-4.0	12

*During the first few hours of life

(con't)

Neonatal Resuscitation (con't)
Fluid (ml/kg/day)

Birth Wt (g)	< 1000	1000 – 1500	> 1500
Day 1	100	80	80
Day 2	140	110	90
Day 3	180	140	120

*If pulmonary edema, ↓ fluid to 50 ml/kg/d
*If < 1300 g give D_5W, if > 1300 g give $D_{10}W$
*Add 0.2 NS on Day 2
*Add KCl 10 mEq/500 ml on Day 3 if UO adequate

Electrolyte Requirements
3 mEq Na^+/100 ml H_2O metabolized
2 mEq Cl^-/100 ml H_2O metabolized
2 mEq K^+/100 ml H_2O metabolized

Hypoglycemia
Premie	< 25 mg/dl
Term < 72 hr	< 35 mg/dl
Term > 72 hr	< 45 mg/dl

*Consider the neonate to be hypoglycemic if the bedside test reads < 50 mg/dl

– – – – – – – – – – – – – – – – – – – –

PEDIATRIC ADVANCED LIFE SUPPORT – OVERVIEW

Tachycardia w/ Poor Perfusion

- QRS ≤ 0.08 sec
  - **Probable ST**
    - P-waves present and wnl
    - Variable R-R w/ constant PR
    - Infants: < 220 bpm
    - Child: 180 bpm
  - Identify and treat cause
    - Fever
    - Shock
    - Pain
    - Hypovolemia
    - Hypoxia
    - Abnormal electrolytes
    - Drug ingestions
    - Pneumothorax
    - Cardiac tamponade

- **Probable SVT**
  - P-waves absent or wnl
  - HR NOT variable w/ activity
  - Abrupt rate Δ's
  - Infants: > 220 bpm
  - Children: > 180 bpm

(con't)

PALS – Probable SVT (con't)
- **Immediate Cardioversion**
  - 0.5 – 1.0 J/kg
    - *May ↑ to 2 J/kg
    - **OR**
  - Adenosine 0.1 mg/kg
    - *Follow w/ rapid 2 – 5 ml NS bolus
    - *May double dose and repeat once as needed
    - *MAX: 12 mg
- Consider alternative medications
  - Amiodarone 5 mg/kg IV over 20 – 60 min
    - **OR**
  - Procainamide 15 mg/kg IV over 30 – 60 min
    - *Ø **administer amiodarone and procainamide together**
- Consult pediatric cardiologist

- **QRS > 0.08 sec (Probable VT)**
  - **Immediate cardioversion**
    - 0.5 – 1.0 J/kg
  - Consider alternative medications
    - Amiodarone 5 mg/kg IV over 20 – 60 min
      - **OR**

- Procainamide 15 mg/kg IV
  over 30 – 60 min
  ***∅ administer amiodarone
  and procainamide together
  OR**
- Lidocaine 1 mg/kg IV bolus
- Consult pediatric cardiologist

Tachycardia w/ Adequate Perfusion
- **QRS ≤ 0.08 sec**
  - **Probable ST**
    - P-waves present and wnl
    - Variable R-R w/ constant PR
    - Infants: < 220 bpm
    - Child: 180 bpm
  - Identify and treat cause
    - Fever
    - Shock
    - Pain
    - Hypovolemia
    - Hypoxia
    - Abnormal electrolytes
    - Drug ingestions
    - Pneumothorax
    - Cardiac tamponade

(con't)

PALS – Tachycardia w/ Adequate Perfusion (con't)

- **Probable SVT**
  - P-waves absent or wnl
  - Abrupt rate Δ to or from wnl
  - Infants: > 220 bpm
  - Children: > 180 bpm
- Consider vagal maneuvers
- Adenosine 0.1 mg/kg
  *Follow w/ rapid 2 – 5 ml NS bolus
  *May double dose and repeat once as needed
  *MAX: 12 mg
- Consult pediatric cardiologist
- Attempt cardioversion w/ 0.5 – 1.0 J/kg
  *May ↑ to 2 J/kg in needed

- **QRS > 0.08 sec (Probable VT)**
  - Identify and treat reversible causes, e.g. electrolyte imbalance, drug toxicity, etc.
  - Consider alternative medications
    - Amiodarone 5 mg/kg IV over 20 – 60 min
      OR
    - Procainamide 15 mg/kg IV over 30 – 60 min
      ∅ administer amiodarone and procainamide together
      OR
    - Lidocaine 1 mg/kg IV bolus

- Consult pediatric cardiologist
- Prepare for cardioversion

Bradycardia w/ Severe Cardiorespiratory Compromise
- ABC's, VS, etc.
- Perform chest compressions if, despite oxygenation and ventilation, HR < 60 in infant or child w/ poor systemic perfusion
- Start IV or IO access
- Epinephrine
  - IV/IO: 0.01 mg/kg (1:10,000, 0.1 ml/kg)
  - ET: 0.1 mg/kg (1:1000, 0.1 ml/kg)
  - Repeat q 3 – 5 min at same dose
- Atropine 0.02 mg/kg
*MR × 1
*Minimum dose: 0.1 mg
*MAX SINGLE DOSE:
  - 0.5 mg for child
  - 1 mg for adolescent
- Consider external or esophageal pacing

(con't)

PALS – (con't)
VF/Pulseless VT
- ABC's
- Defibrillate 2 J/kg, 4 J/kg, 4 J/kg
- ETT / IV / IO if not already established
- Epinephrine q 3 – 5 min
    - IV/IO: 0.01 mg/kg
             (1:10,000, 0.1 ml/kg)
    - ET: 0.1 mg/kg (1:1000, 0.1 ml/kg)
- Defibrillate 4 J/kg 30 – 60 sec after each medication
- Antiarrhythmics
    - Amiodarone 5 mg/kg IV/IO
      MAX: 15 mg/kg/d
              OR
    - Lidocaine 1 mg/kg IV/IO
      MAX: 3 mg/kg
              OR
    - Magnesium 25 – 50 mg/kg IV/IO for Torsades de Pointes or hypomagnesemia
      MAX: 2 g
- Defibrillate 4 J/kg

Asystole / Pulseless Electrical Activity
- ABC's
- Identify and treat cause
  - Hypovolemia
  - Hypoxemia
  - Hypothermia
  - Hyper-/hypokalemia and metabolic disorders
  - Tamponade
  - Tension pneumothorax
  - Toxins/poisons/drugs
  - Thromboembolism
- Epinephrine q 3 – 5 min
  - IV/IO: 0.01 mg/kg (1:10,000, 0.1 ml/kg)
  - ET: 0.1 mg/kg (1:1000, 0.1 ml/kg)

- -

PEDIATRIC VITAL SIGN AND REFERENCE

Age	Kg Wt	SBP	HR	RR	ETT	NG
0-2 mo	3.5	70	135	35	3.5	8F
3 mo	6	80	125	28	3.5	8F
6 mo	8	90	125	24	4.0	10F
1 yr	10	95	110	22	4.0	10F
2 yr	12.5	95	110	18	4.5	12F
3 yr	14.5	95	100	16	5.0	12F
4 yr	17	95	100	14	5.0	14F
5 yr	18.5	100	95	14	5.5	14F
6 yr	21	105	90	12	5.5	14F
7 yr	23	105	90	12	5.5	14F
8 yr	25	105	90	12	6.0	16F
9 yr	28	110	85	12	6.0	16F

*Kg wt:
- 1 yr = 10 kg
- Add 2 kg for each additional year

*Patient is hypotensive if:
BP $\leq 70 + (2 \times$ age in years)

*Mean SBP > 2 yo:
$90 + (2 \times$ age in years)

*Mean DBP:
$0.66 \times$ SBP for age

*Neonates MAP should approximate its gestational age
*Term neonate hypotensive if SBP < 60 mmHg

*Sinus Tachycardia if:
- < 3 mo HR > 200
- 3 mo – 2 yr HR > 190
- 2 – 10 yr HR > 140

TETRALOGY OF FALLOT

- Obstruction of right ventricular outflow:
    - Pulmonary stenosis
    - Right ventricular infundibulum
- Right ventricular hypertrophy
- Dextroposition of the aorta with septal override
- Ventricular septal defect

*The degree of cyanosis is directly proportional of the severity of the pulmonary stenosis

*CXR: Boot shaped heart w/ ↓ pulmonary markings

Hypercyanotic Spells

- Sudden onset of cyanosis
- Dyspnea
- Alterations in consciousness
- ↓ intensity of systolic murmur

↑ R to L shunt ↓ pulmonary blood flow. The patient's restlessness and agitation leads to crying and ↑ pulmonary vascular resistance which leads to ↓ pulmonary blood flow and hypoxemia. ↑ hypoxemia leads to acidosis which causes pulmonary vasoconstriction and ↓ pulmonary blood flow which all leads to ↑ hypoxemia and the cycle repeats itself.

*Age: 1 mo – 12 yrs
*Peak: 1 – 3 mo
*More frequent in the morning upon awakening

Tx:

- Comfort the child and place the child in the knee-chest position
- O$_2$ via face mask
- Morphine 0.1 – 0.2 mg/kg SC if IV not available
- IV fluid replacement or volume expansion; if anemic give blood
- NaHCO$_3$ 0.5 – 1.0 mEq/kg IV for acidosis
- Repeat morphine 0.01 – 0.1 mg/kg IV
- Consider
  - Propranolol 0.05 – 0.1 mg/kg IV
    MAX: 1 mg/dose
    *Consult w/ pediatric cardiology and cardiothoracic surgery before administration
  - Esmolol 500 – 1000 µg/kg IV followed by an infusion of 100 – 300 µg/kg/min
  - Phenylephrine 10 – 50 µg/kg/min bolus
    *MR and double dose to a maximum total bolus of 50 µg/kg/min
    *Infuse 1 – 10 µg/kg/min
- Consider general anesthesia

- -

TOTAL PARENTRAL NUTRITION

Requirements:

- Fluid/Calories:

0 – 10 kg	100 ml or Cal/kg/d
10 – 20 kg	50 ml or Cal/kg/d
> 20 kg	10 ml or Cal/kg/d

- Protein: 1.0 – 2.5 g/kg/d

- Lipids: 1 wk – 2 yrs: 1 – 4 Gm/kg/d
  > 2 yrs: 1 – 3 Gm/kg/d

- Electrolytes
  - Na^+ 2 – 4 mEq/100 ml H_2O metabolized
  - Cl^- 2 – 3 mEq/100 ml H_2O metabolized
  - K^+ 2 – 3 mEq/100 ml H_2O metabolized

  *Usually added as a fixed amount w/ the other electrolytes

  *Acetate will cause alkalosis – good to use if patient has metabolic acidosis

  *If use > 20 mEq KPO_4 and > 20 mEq Ca^{++} gluconate, add L-cysteine to ↓ the pH of the solution to prevent precipitation

Laboratory Studies:
- Glucose q 6 hr w/ coverage
  *Can add insulin to the TPN
- Daily: Electrolytes, Ca^{++}, Mg^{++}, HPO_4^-,
  CBC, BUN and Cr until stable,
  then q 3 d
- Daily: Weights and I & O's
- Weekly: LFT's, TG, PT/PTT, prealbumin,
  albumin

CALCULATIONS:

Amino Acids:
- 1.5%   provides 0.06 kcal/ml
- 2.0%   provides 0.08 kcal/ml
- 2.5%   provides 0.10 kcal/ml
- 4.25% provides 0.17 kcal/ml

Dextrose:
- 10%   provides 0.34 kcal/ml
- 12.5% provides 0.43 kcal/ml
- 15%   provides 0.51 kcal/ml
- 25%   provides 0.85 kcal/ml

Intravenous Fat Emulsion:
- 10% provides 1.1 kcal/ml
- 20% provides 2.0 kcal/ml

(con't)

TPN (con't)
FLUID CALCULATIONS:
Step 1:
Pt wt_____ kg × _____ml/kg/d = _____total
volume

Step 2:
_____total volume − _____ml lipid/d = _____ml
dextrose − AA solution volume/d

Step 3:
Total Volume ÷ 24 hr = _____ml/hr to infuse

CALORIE CALCULATIONS:
Dextrose sol'n: ___kcal/ml × ___ml = ___kcal
+
*From step 2 above

AA sol'n: ___kcal/ml × ___ml = ___kcal
+

IV Fat sol'n: ___kcal/ml × ___ml = ___kcal
=

             TOTAL = _____ kcal//d

             TOTAL ÷ kg wt = _____kcal/kg
- - - - - - - - - - - - - - - - - - - -

304

ACID-BASE ANALYSIS – STEPS TO THE APPROACH OF

1. Determine whether the 1° disturbance is an acidemia (pH < 7.35) or an alkalemia (pH > 7.45)
2. Determine whether the 1° disturbance is a respiratory or a metabolic problem
   - If acidemic
     - Respiratory acidosis: $PaCO_2 > 45$
     - Metabolic acidosis: $HCO_3^- < 22$

   - If alkalemic
     - Respiratory alkalosis: $PaCO_2 < 35$
     - Metabolic alkalosis: $HCO_3^- > 26$
3. Determine the anion gap
4. Determine the corrected serum bicarbonate
5. Determine whether the degree of compensation is appropriate in metabolic disturbances or whether the disorder is acute or chronic in respiratory disorders

*For above calculations, see Arterial Blood Gases

- -

ADULT RESPIRATORY DISTRESS SYNDROME

Diffuse inflammatory process involving both lungs believed to originate from the systemic activation of neutrophils

Causes: Sepsis, multiple transfusions, pulmonary contusion, aspiration of gastric contents, multiple fractures, drug OD

S/S: Tachypnea, progressive hypoxemia refractory to O_2, bilateral pulmonary infiltrates within 24 hr (may be more prominent in the periphery)

CLINICAL CRITERIA
1. Acute onset
2. Patient has a predisposing condition to ARDS
3. $P_{AO_2}/F_{IO_2} < 200$ mmHg regardless of amount of PEEP
4. Bilateral infiltrates on CXR
5. PCWP ≤ 18 mmHg

*Pneumonia, acute pulmonary embolism and cardiogenic pulmonary edema may mimic ARDS

Tx:
- Ventilator
  - V_T 7 – 10 ml/kg
  - PIP < 35 cm H_2O
  - F_{IO_2} < 60%
  - PEEP 5 – 10 cm H_2O to keep
    SaO_2 > 90%

- Tissue Oxygenation
  - V_{O_2} < 100 ml/min/m^2
  - Lactic acid level < 4 mmol/L

- Cardiovascular
  - wnl CVP and PCWP
  - Hgb > 10 g/dl
  - CI > 3 L/min/m^2
    *If unable to use fluids, dobutamine
    is preferred over dopamine since
    dopamine causes vasoconstriction
    of the pulmonary vasculature

- -

ALVEOLAR – ARTERIAL GAS PRESSURE DIFFERENCE (A:a DO₂)

Difference between the measured partial pressure of a gas in the alveoli and the simultaneously measured partial pressure of that gas in systemic arterial blood. Difference may indicate a functional abnormality in pulmonary gas exchange, i.e. V/Q mismatch, R → L shunt.

FORMULA:

$$A:a\ DO_2 = (760\ mmHg - 47\ mmHg) \times FiO_2 - (PaCO_2 / 0.8) - PaO_2$$

760 mmHg: atmospheric pressure
47 mmHg: partial pressure of H_2O at 100% saturation
0.21: F_iO_2 of room air
0.8: conversion factor for respiratory quotient (can also multiply the $PaCO_2$ by 1.25 instead of dividing by 0.8)
PaO_2: as measured from the ABG

If on room air: $150 - (PaCO_2 / 0.8) - PaO_2$

WNL: 10 – 20 on room air
   *Indicates that the lung parenchyma is normal

308

*Add 5 – 7 for q 10% ↑ in FiO_2

*If FiO_2 1.0 then the A-a gradient
  should be < 50

*Upper limit wnl for age: $0.3 \times age$

*↑ gradients are seen w/ mucous plugging,
bronchospasm, asthma, COPD, atrial septal
defect, pneumothorax, pulmonary emboli,
atelectasis, pneumonia

A/a ratio = $\dfrac{P_aO_2}{150 - (P_aCO_2 / 0.8)}$

wnl < 10 on room air or <100 on 100% O_2

*If patient is receiving 100% O_2 and P_aO_2 is
not > 600, then a shunt exists

- -

ARTERIAL BLOOD GASES

Golden Rule I: An ↑ in $PaCO_2$ by 10 torr ↑ the pH by 0.1, and vise versa

Golden Rule II: pH Δ of 0.15 = base Δ of 10 mEq/L

Quick Method (gives general condition)

DISORDER	pH	PCO₂	HCO₃
RESP ACID	↓	↑	N
RESP ALKA	↑	↓	N
META ACID	↓	N	↓
META ALKA	↑	N	↑
COMP RESP ACID	N↓	↑	↑
COMP RESP ALKA	N↑	↓	↓
COMP META ACID	N↓	↓	↓
COMP META ALKA	N↑	↑	↑

Metabolic Acidosis

- $PaCO_2 = (1.5 \times HCO_3) + 8.4$ if adequate compensation is present
  *$PaCO_2$ = last two digits of pH
- If $PaCO_2$ > expected, respiratory acidosis is also present
- If $PaCO_2$ < expected, respiratory alkalosis is also present

*2.5 mEq/L $NaHCO_3$ × kg wt infused over ½ hr will ↑ the serum bicarbonate level by 5 mEq/L

Metabolic Alkalosis

- An $\uparrow$ in HCO_3 by 10 will $\uparrow$ the pH by 0.15 and the $PaCO_2$ by 7 (Golden Rule II)
- If $PaCO_2 > 50$, a 1° respiratory acidosis is also present
- If $PaCO_2 < 40$, a 1° respiratory alkalosis is also present

*Respiratory compensation will not $\uparrow$ the $PaCO_2 > 50$

Respiratory Acidosis

- For the acute patient an $\uparrow$ in $PaCO_2$ by 10 will $\downarrow$ the pH by 0.1 and $\uparrow$ the HCO_3 by 1.0 (Golden Rule I)
- Expected $\downarrow$ in pH = $\dfrac{0.08 \times (PaCO_2 - 40)}{10}$

- For the chronic patient an $\uparrow$ in $PaCO_2$ by 10 will $\downarrow$ the pH by 0.03 and will $\uparrow$ the HCO_3 by 3.5
- Expected $\downarrow$ in pH = $\dfrac{0.03 \times (PaCO_2 - 40)}{10}$

(con't)

Arterial Blood Gases (con't)
Respiratory Alkalosis

- For the acute patient a $\downarrow$ in $PaCO_2$ by 10 will $\uparrow$ the pH by 0.1 and $\downarrow$ the HCO_3 by 2.5

- Expected $\downarrow$ in pH = $\dfrac{0.08 \times (PaCO_2 - 40)}{10}$

- For the chronic patient a $\downarrow$ in $PaCO_2$ by 10 will $\uparrow$ the pH by 0.03 and $\downarrow$ the HCO_3 by 5

- Expected $\downarrow$ in pH = $\dfrac{0.03 \times (PaCO_2 - 40)}{10}$

Normal Values

BLOOD	pH	pCO₂	PO₂	HCO₃
Arterial < 1 yo	7.33 – 7.40	35 – 45	80 – 100	23 – 27
Arterial > 1 yo	7.35 – 7.45	35 – 45	80 – 100	23 – 27
Venous	7.35 – 7.40	45 – 50	30 – 50	24 – 29

Arterial Blood Gases In Asthma

	PaO₂	PaCO₂	pH
Mild	wnl	$\downarrow$	> 7.45
Moderate	sl $\downarrow$	mod $\downarrow$	> 7.45
Severe	mod $\downarrow$	wnl	wnl
Failure	markedly $\downarrow$	$\uparrow$	< 7.35

ETCO₂ : $35 - 45$ mmHg
*End-Tidal CO_2 is normally within 3 mmHg of
the $PaCO_2$

    ↑: Hypoventilation, $NaHCO_3$
    administration, hyperthermia, ↑ blood
    flow to the lungs (s/p resuscitation,
    improvement of hypotension, H_2O in
    capnograph head

    ↓: Hyperventilation, hypothermia,
    pulmonary edema, air embolism,
    ↓ blood flow to the lungs, pulmonary
    embolism, migration of the ETT into
    the mainstem bronchus

*1% $EtCO_2$ = 7.6 mmHg

- -

POSITIVE PRESSURE VENTILATION

Initiating Volume Ventilation

- Select tidal volume (V_T): 8 – 12 ml/kg
- Select FiO_2: usually start at 1.0
    - ↓ to maintain a PaO_2 > 70 torr on an FiO_2 of < 0.5 – 0.6
- Select rate: normal respiratory rate for age
    - Adjust rate and/or V_T to maintain $PaCO_2$ 35 – 45 torr
- Select inspiratory time (I/E ratio): normally 1:2
    *In obstructive lung diseases: use a prolonged expiratory time and avoid a prolonged inspiratory time
- Select PEEP: physiologic PEEP is 5 cm H_2O
    - Can be adjusted up to 15 cm H_2O
    - Monitor hemodynamic effects and status of patient
    - Goal is to maintain a PaO_2 > 70 torr
- Assess for adequate ventilation and oxygenation: chest excursion, breath sounds, SaO_2, color, hypotension, chest x-ray for ETT tube placement and lung inflation, ABG

- Plateau pressure ($P_{plateau}$) should be < 30 cm H_2O, if > 30, ↓ RR
  - ↑ P_{peak} w/ wnl $P_{plateau}$ indicates ↑ airway resistance, i.e. obstructed ETT, airway obstruction from secretions, acute bronchospasm
  - ↑ P_{peak} w/ ↑ $P_{plateau}$ indicates ↓ distensibility of the lung and chest wall, i.e. pneumothorax, lobar atelectasis, acute pulmonary edema, worsening pneumonia or ARDS, ↑ auto-PEEP

Initiating Pressure Ventilation
- Start at a positive inspiratory pressure (PIP) of 20 cm H_2O
- Start w/ a PEEP of 5 cm H_2O
- Select rate: normal respiratory rate for age
- Select FiO_2: < 0.5 – 0.6 to prevent O_2 toxicity
- Assess for adequate ventilation and oxygenation: chest excursion, breath sounds, SaO_2, color, chest x-ray for ETT placement and lung inflation, ABG

(con't)

Positive Pressure Ventilation (con't)
Basic Ventilation Management

1. To $\uparrow$ PaO_2:
   - $\uparrow$ FiO_2
   - $\uparrow$ PEEP
   - $\uparrow$ minute ventilation – also $\downarrow$ CO_2
   - $\uparrow$ mean airway pressure (P_{aw}) – usually > 30 cm H_2O is not necessary
   - Diuresis, suction, respiratory treatment

2. To $\downarrow$ PaO_2:
   - $\downarrow$ any parameter in #1

3. To $\uparrow$ $PaCO_2$:
   - $\downarrow$ minute ventilation

4. To $\downarrow$ $PaCO_2$:
   - $\uparrow$ minute ventilation
   - $\uparrow$ PEEP in worsening lung dz
   - $\downarrow$ PEEP in recovery phase

Lung Protective
Use: ARDS

V_T:	5 – 10 ml/kg
$P_{Plateau}$:	< 32 cm H_2O
PEEP:	5 – 15 cm H_2O
ABG:	pH = 7.20 – 7.44 (permissive hypercarbia)

Discontinuing Positive Pressure Ventilation

- Determine why the patient needed positive pressure ventilation and whether or not this condition has resolved
- Is the patient awake and following commands? – not necessary but helpful.
- Discontinue sedation and paralytics
- Assess the patient for anything that would cause a failure of extubation, i.e. fever, abdominal distention, malnutrition, etc.
- Discontinue feedings 2 – 3 hours prior to extubation or apply suction to NG tube to prevent aspiration
- Wean FiO_2 to ≤ 0.4
- Wean SIMV to 2 – 4 breaths/min in infants, CPAP of 5 cm H_2O w/ PPS of 5 cm H_2O in children and adults
- Wean PEEP to 2 – 3 cm H_2O in infants, 5 cm H_2O in children and adults and 8 cm H_2O in patients w/ COPD
- Discontinue Support when:
  - $V_T > 5 – 7$ ml/kg
  - $RR/V_T < 105$
  - Minute ventilation < 12
  - PEEP ≤ 5 – 8 cm H_2O
  - FiO_2 ≤ 0.4
  - $PaO_2 > 60$ torr
  - RR < 25 – 30
  - pH > 7.35

PULMONARY EMBOLISM

Predisposing Factors:
- Prolonged immobilization
- Surgery within 3 months
- History of DVT or PE
- Trauma/Burns
- Pregnancy
- Malignancy
- Hypercoagulable states

S/S
- Dyspnea – most common symptom
- Chest pain – usually pleuritic in nature secondary pulmonary infarction
- Respiratory rate > 16
- Apprehension – secondary to hypoxia
- Rales

Dx:
- ↑ A:a gradient

- ECG changes
  - Sinus tachycardia – most common finding
  - Tall P-wave in inferior leads (R atrial overload)
  - S_I, Q_{III}, $\perp_{III}$: S-wave in Lead I, Q-wave in Lead III, T-wave inversion in Lead III
  - S_I, S_{II}, S_{III}: S-wave in Lead I, S-wave in Lead II, S-wave in Lead III

- CXR
  - Hampton's Hump:
    - Pleural density or lung consolidation w/ rounded borders that point toward the hilus
  - Westermark Sign:
    - Dilated pulmonary outflow tract on the side of the pulmonary embolus. There will be an area of decreased perfusion distal to the blockage.

- Venous duplex ultrasound

- Ventilation/Perfusion Lung Scan
  - Normal:
    - Presence of a clinically significant PE is excluded
  - Low Probability:
    - ∅ reliably exclude a PE in patients w/ cardiovascular dz
    - If combined w/ (−) evaluation for leg vein thrombosis − probably safe to observe
  - Intermediate Probability:
    - NO diagnostic value
  - High Probability:
    - 85% chance of having a PE

(con't)

Pulmonary Embolus – Dx (con't)

- Pulmonary Angiography
  *GOLD STANDARD

- D-dimer – role still being evaluated

Tx:
- ABC's
- IV fluids if ↓ CVP
- Dopamine if wnl or ↑ CVP
- Heparin bolus of 10,000 – 20,000 U
  followed by an infusion of 1000 U/hr
  *Heparin ∅ cross the placenta –
  therefore it is safe in pregnancy
- Thrombolytic therapy for:
  - Hemodynamically unstable patients
  - Persistent hypotension despite
    appropriate medical management
  *NOT proven to ↓ morbidity or mortality
- Surgical embolectomy

- -

RAPID SEQUENCE INTUBATION

1. Lidocaine 1.5 mg/kg IV (especially in head injured patients)
2. Etomidate 0.3 mg/kg IV for adults and children > 10 yo
3. Intubation attempt. If unsuccessful proceed w/ paralytics.
4. Defasiculating dose of vecuronium 1 mg IV in adults. Peds dose 0.01 mg/kg (1 mg MAX).
   *Skip in children under 4 years of age
5. Atropine 0.01 – 0.02 mg/kg IV
   *Minimum 0.2 mg; MAX 1 mg
   *Use only in children less than 5 years of age
6. Succinylcholine 1.5 mg/kg IV – adult; 2 mg/kg IV – peds; administer within seconds of vecuronium dose
   *If second dose of succinylcholine is needed, administer atropine in both adults and children
7. Wait 60 seconds and attempt intubation

*For sedation may use:
- Midazolam 2 – 4 mg in 2 mg increments IV in adults and 0.1 mg/kg (2 mg MAX) in children
- Fentanyl 2 µg/kg slow IV
- Ketamine 2 mg/kg in adults and 1 mg/kg in children
  *Bronchodilates, ↑ BP

(con't)

Rapid Sequence Intubation (con't)

Effects of medications used in RSI:

- Lidocaine 1.5 mg/kg
    - Blunts the ↑ in ICP
    - Suppresses the cough reflex
    - Attenuates the ↑ in airway resistance
- $1/10^{th}$ the paralyzing dose of a nondepolarizing NMB
    - Blunts the response of ↑ ICP due to succinylcholine
- Atropine 0.01 – 0.02 mg/kg
    - Blocks the ↑ vagal stimulation of the SA node response in children that occurs during laryngoscopy which leads to bradycardia
- Fentanyl 2 µg/kg over 1 min
    - Mitigates the Reflex Sympathetic Response to Laryngoscopy
- Ketamine 2 mg/kg in the adult or 1 mg/kg in the child
    - Causes bronchodilation – good if patient is having bronchospasm
    - ↑ the blood pressure – good if patient is hypotensive

- -

ACETAMINOPHEN OVERDOSE

S/S: Anorexia, vomiting, diaphoresis

- Hepatic enzymes begin to rise 24 – 36 hr post ingestion
- AST peaks earliest @ 72 – 96 hr
- Minimal dose of APAP capable of causing liver toxicity:
    - 140 mg/kg in children
    - 7.5 g in adults

STAGES:

I:	1/2 – 24 hr:	Anorexia, N/V, malaise, pallor, diaphoresis
II:	24 – 48 hr:	Abdominal pain, liver tenderness, ↑ hepatic enzymes, oliguria
III:	72 – 96 hr:	Peak hepatic enzymes, ↑ bilirubin level, ↑ PT
IV:	4 days – 2 wks:	Resolution of hepatotoxicity or progressive hepatic failure

*Rumack-Matthew Nomogram starts at 4 hr post ingestion. It ∅ provide useful information when there is chronic ingestion or an acute ingestion of sustained release preparations.

(con't)

Acetaminophen Overdose (con't)

Tx: Adult/Peds
- Baseline Labs: AST, ALT, bilirubin, BUN, PT
- Gastric lavage if patient presents within 4 hr of ingestion
- Activated charcoal w/ sorbitol if patient presents within 4 hr of ingestion
    - Adult: 50 – 60 g
    - Peds: 1 g/kg
- N-acetylcysteine
  *See acetylcysteine dosing p. 90 – 91
- Droperidol or metoclopramide for N/V

- -

BENZODIAZEPINE OVERDOSE

S/S: Hypotension, dizziness, ataxia, altered mental status, slurred speech, respiratory depression, coma

Tx: Adult/Peds
- ABC's
- Gastric lavage
- Activated charcoal w/ sorbitol
    - Adult: 50 – 60 g
    - Peds: 1 g/kg
- Flumazenil
    - Adult:
        - 0.2 mg IV over 15 sec, then
        - 0.3 mg @ 1-minute intervals to a maximum total dose of 3 mg

324

- If a partial response is seen additional incremental doses of 0.5 mg may be given to a maximum of 5 mg
- Recurrence of sedation or respiratory depression can be treated as above or with a continuous infusion of 0.1 – 0.5 mg/hr

- Peds:
  - Initial dose 0.01 mg/kg MAX: 0.2 mg
  - Then, 0.005 – 0.01 mg/kg (MAX: 0.2 mg) given q 1 min to a maximum total cumulative dose of 1 mg
    *Doses may be repeated in 20 min up to a maximum of 3 mg in 1 hr

*∅ use if patient has taken a mixed overdose
*Difficult to control sz may occur

- - - - - - - - - - - - - - - - - - - -

BETA BLOCKER OVERDOSE

S/S: Bradycardia, AV block, hypotension,
CHF, altered mental status, coma, sz,
hypoventilation, bronchospasm,
hypoglycemia, mesenteric ischemia

Tx: Adult/Peds
- ABC's
- Gastric lavage
- ∅ **give ipecac** – may cause
cardiovascular collapse due to vagal
stimulation from vomiting
- Activated charcoal w/ sorbitol
  - Adult: 50 – 60 g
  - Peds: 1 g/kg
- Atropine for vagally induced bradycardia
  - Adult/Peds: MAX: 0.03 mg/kg
- NS boluses for hypotension
  - Adult/Peds: 20 ml/kg
- Pacing, either TVP or TCP
- Glucagon for bradycardia and
hypotension
  - Adult/Peds: 50 – 150 µg/kg
- Glucagon gtt for bradycardia and
hypotension
  - Adult/Peds: 1 – 5 mg/hr titrated to
patient response
- Isoproterenol for bradycardia
  - Adult: 2 – 200 µg/min
  - Peds: 0.1 – 2.0 µg/kg/min

- Norepinephrine for hypotension
  - Adult: 2 – 12 µg/min
  - Peds: 0.05 – 2.0 µg/kg/min
- Epinephrine gtt for hypotension
  - Adult/Peds: 0.1 – 1.5 µg/kg/min
  *Use w/ caution – may cause HTN w/ reflexive bradycardia
- CaCl 10% sol'n for continued hypotension
  - Adult: 5 – 20 ml IV
  - Peds: 10 – 25 mg/kg IV
  *Ca gluconate is preferred if the patient is extremely acidotic
- Consider dobutamine
- Bronchospasm: Theophylline
- Sz: Benzodiazepines and phenytoin
- Dialysis is useful for nadolol, sotalol, atenolol and acebutolol

- - - - - - - - - - - - - - - - - -

CALCIUM CHANNEL BLOCKER OVERDOSE

S/S: Hypotension, altered mental status, coma, sz, bradycardia, AV block, reflex tachycardia, asystole, pulmonary edema, hypocalcemia, hyperglycemia

Tx: Adult/Peds
- ABC's
- Gastric lavage
- NS boluses for hypotension
  - Adult/Peds: 20 mg/kg
- Dopamine for hypotension
  - Adult/Peds: 2 – 20 µg/kg/min
- CaCl 10% sol'n for hypotension, bradycardia, heart block
  - Adult: 10 – 20 ml
  - Peds: 10 – 25 mg/kg
  *Ca gluconate is preferred if the patient is extremely acidotic
  *MR × 3 – 4 doses
- Epinephrine gtt
  - Adult/Peds: 0.1 – 1.5 µg/kg/min
- Glucagon for bradycardia and hypotension
  - Adult/Peds: 50 – 150 µg/kg
- Glucagon gtt for bradycardia and hypotension
  - Adult/Peds: 1 – 5 mg/hr titrated to patient response
- For continued hypotension consider MAST and IABP

- Atropine for bradycardia
  - Adult/Peds: MAX 0.03 mg/kg
- Pacing, either TVP or TCP
- Sz: Benzodiazepines and phenytoin
- Hemodialysis is NOT helpful

- - - - - - - - - - - - - - - - - - - -

CARBON MONOXIDE POISONING

S/S: see chart below

- CO affinity for Hgb is 200 times greater than O_2
- Half-life on room air is 4 – 5 hr
- Half-life ↓ to 1.5 hr on 100% O_2
- Half-life ↓ to 23 min w/ HBO therapy @ 3 atm

Tx: Adult/Peds
- 100% O_2/NRB
- Measure CoHb q 2 – 4 hr
- Continue O_2 until blood levels are < 10%

Admit:
- COHb > 25% or COHb > 15% in patient w/ CAD
- Acute ECG changes
- Abnormal neuropsychiatric evaluation
- Metabolic acidosis associated w/ CO inhalation

(con't)

Carbon Monoxide Poisoning (con't)
Admit (con't)
- Abnormal thermoregulation
- PO_2 < 60 mmHg
- Pregnant patient w/ sx or COHb > 10%

HBO Rx: CO > 25% or symptomatic patient

S/S: 0 – 10 None
10 – 20 Slight HA, dyspnea w/ vigorous
exertion, may be asymptomatic
20 – 30 Throbbing HA, dyspnea w/
moderate exertion, N/V,
↓ judgement
30 – 40 Severe HA, N/V, visual
disturbances, tachycardia,
hyperpnea, hypotension,
confusion
40 – 50 Syncope, tachycardia,
tachypnea
50 – 60 Coma, convulsions, Cheynne-
Stokes respirations
60 – 70 Compensated cardiorespiratory
function, convulsions,
respiratory arrest, death
80 – 90 Death

- - - - - - - - - - - - - - - - - - - -

COCAINE OVERDOSE

Stimulates release and blocks the reuptake of norepinephrine, epinephrine, dopamine, and serotonin causing HTN, tachycardia, euphoria

β effects: tachycardia, (+) inotropy
α effects: ↓ coronary blood flow, induces coronary artery vasospasm

Tx: Adults:
   PSVT (hemodynamically stable):
   - O_2
   - Diazepam 5 – 20 mg IV over 5 – 20 min

   VT (hemodynamically stable):
   - O_2
   - Lidocaine 1 – 1.5 mg/kg*
     *Increase risk of sz due to the synergistic toxic effects of lidocaine and cocaine
   - Escalating dose of diazepam 5 – 20 mg
   - Propranolol 0.5 – 1.0 mg q 5 min or labetalol (α and β effects) 20 mg IV over 2 min
     *MR 40 – 80 mg q 10 min
     *MAX DOSE: 300 mg

(con't)

331

Cocaine Overdose (con't)
VF:
- Defib 200 J, 300 J, 360 J
- O_2, hyperventilation
- Epinephrine 1.0 mg – single dose only, followed by defibrillation
  *Limit epinephrine to 1.0 mg q 5 – 10 min if needed
  *∅ use high dose epinephrine
- Lidocaine 1.5 mg/kg, defibrillation
  *Avoid repeated doses
- Propranolol 1.0 mg q 1 min
  *MAX DOSE: 3 – 5 mg
- Defib after each dose of propranolol
- Try Mg^{++}, procainamide, bretylium

CP/AMI:
- O_2
- ASA 325 mg
- Nitrates
- Benzodiazepines
- Magnesium
- Morphine

*∅ use β-blockers, may cause vasospasm
*tPA is not routinely used. AMI is usually
caused by vasospasm not thrombus
formation. Check cardiac enzymes or take
the patient to the cardiac catheterization lab.
*∅ use haloperidol for sedation – ↓ sz
threshold

- - - - - - - - - - - - - - - - - - - -

CYANIDE TOXICITY

S/S: Disorientation, agitation, lethargy, sz,
coma, cerebral death, initial ↑ HR and
BP followed by ↓ BP, shock and lethal
cardiac arrhythmias, early tachypnea
followed by apnea, N/V, severe
metabolic acidosis
*NO cyanosis is seen

Tx: Adult:
- Amyl nitrate 0.3 ml by inhalation for
15 – 30 sec q 1 min followed by
- Na^+ nitrite 300 mg (10 ml of 3% sol'n) IV
slowly over 2 – 4 min followed
immediately by
*MR 150 mg in 2 hr if persistent or
recurrent signs of toxicity occur
- Na^+ thiosulfate 12.5 g (50 ml of 25%
sol'n) IV over 10 min
*MR 6.25 g in 2 hr if persistent or
recurrent signs of toxicity occur

- - - - - - - - - - - - - - - - - - - -

DRUG LEVELS – BLOOD

Drug	Therapeutic	Toxic
APAP	1 – 30 µg/ml	> 200
Amikacin		
Peak 20 – 30 µg/ml		
Trough < 10 µg/ml		
Amiodarone	2.5 – 6.7 µg/ml	
Amitriptyline	100 – 250 mg/ml	> 500
Carbamazepine	4 – 12 µg/ml	> 15
Chlordiazepoxide	700 – 1000 ng/ml	> 5000
Disopyramide	variable	> 7
Diazepam	100 – 1000 ng/ml	> 5000
Digoxin	0.8 – 2.0 ng/ml	> 25
EtOH	100 mg/ml	> 400
Gentamycin		
Peak 5 – 10 µg/ml		
Trough < 2 µg/ml		
Imipramine	125 – 250 ng/ml	> 500
Lithium	0.6 – 1.2 mEq/L	> 2
Lidocaine	1.5 – 6.0 µg/ml	> 6 – 8

Drug	Therapeutic	Toxic
N-Acetylprocainamide	5 – 30 mg/L	> 30

*If procainamide + NAPA > 30 = toxic

Phenobarbital	15 – 40 g/ml	35 – 80
Phenytoin	10 – 20 g/ml	varies w/ sx
Primidone	5 – 12 µg/ml	
Procainamide	4 – 10 g/ml	10 – 12

*If procainamide + NAPA > 30 = toxic

Propranolol	50 – 100 ng/ml	not defined
Quinidine	2 – 5 µg/ml	> 5
Salicylate	< 100 µg/ml	> 100
Theophylline	8 – 12 µg/ml	> 20

* > 16 ↓ inflammation and bronchoconstriction –
occurs in a few days

Thiocyanate	< 10 mg/dl	> 10

Tobramycin
Peak 6 – 10 µg/ml
Trough 2 – 8 µg/ml

Valproic Acid	50 – 100 µg/ml	> 100

Vancomycin
Peak 25 – 40 µg/ml
Trough < 5 – 10

- - - - - - - - - - - - - - - - - - -

ETHYLENE GLYCOL INGESTION

*Commonly used in antifreeze and windshield de-icer fluids

S/S: EtOH inebriation, sz, metabolic acidosis, ataxia, coma, N/V

Tx: Adult/Peds
- ABC's
- Lavage if within 30 min of ingestion
- EtOH rx w/ 10% sol'n if ethylene glycol level > 20 mg/dl, or suspicion of ethylene glycol ingestion while awaiting levels
    - Adult:
        - Load 7.6 – 10 ml/kg IV over 30 min
        - Maintenance: 1.4 – 3 ml/kg/hr
          *GOAL: EtOH level 100 – 150 mg/dl
    - Peds:
        - Load 100% EtOH at 800 mg/kg IV or PO
        - Maintenance: 130 mg/kg/hr
          *GOAL: EtOH level 100 – 150 mg/dl
- Metabolic Acidosis
    - Adult/Peds: NaHCO₃ 1– 3 mEq/kg titrated to a wnl pH
- Pyridoxine (Vitamin B₆)
    - Adult: 100 mg IV qd
    - Peds: 1 – 2 mg/kg/d

Ethylene Glycol Ingestion (con't)
- Thiamine (Vitamin B$_1$)
    - Adult: 100 mg IV qd
    - Peds: 25 mg IV qd
- Dialysis is highly effective
- 4-Methylpyrazole
    - Adult: Load: 15 mg/kg IV
        Maintenance: 10 mg/kg IV q
        12 hr × 4
        doses

*Lethal dose is 2 mg/kg
*Half-life 3 hr
*Metabolite of ethylene glycol, glycolic acid, causes metabolic acidosis, is toxic, and has a half-life of 12 hr
*Oxalic acid binds w/ Ca^{++} causing hypocalcemia

- - - - - - - - - - - - - - - - - - -

METHANOL OVERDOSE
*Commonly used in antifreeze and windshield de-icer fluids

S/S: Altered mental status, HA, visual disturbances, N/V, abdominal pain, tachypnea, respiratory failure

Tx: Adult/Peds
- ABC's
- Lavage if within 30 min of ingestion
(con't)

Methanol Overdose (con't)

- Activated charcoal w/ sorbitol
  - Adult: 50 – 60 g
  - Peds: 1 g/kg
- Folinic acid (Leucovorin)
  - Adult: 1 mg/kg
    - *MAX: 50 mg
- Folic acid
  - Adult: 1 mg/kg IV q 4 hr × 6 doses
- 4-Methylpyrazole
  - Adult: Load: 15 mg/kg IV
    - Maintenance: 10 mg/kg IV q 12 hr × 4 doses
- EtOH rx w/ 10% sol'n if ethylene glycol level > 20 mg/dl, or suspicion of ethylene glycol ingestion while awaiting levels
  - Adult:
    - Load 7.6 – 10 ml/kg IV over 30 min
    - Maintenance: 1.4 – 3 ml/kg/hr
      - *GOAL: EtOH level 100 – 150 mg/dl
  - Peds:
    - Load 100% EtOH at 800 mg/kg IV or PO
    - Maintenance: 130 mg/kg/hr
      - *GOAL: EtOH level 100 – 150 mg/dl
- Hemodialysis for MeOH level > 50 mg/dl, severe acidosis, renal failure or visual disturbances

- - - - - - - - - - - - - - - - - - -

SALICYLATE TOXICITY

S/S:
- 150 mg/kg or less: No significant toxicity: N/V
- 150 – 300 mg/kg: Mild/moderate toxicity: hyperpnea, N/V, diaphoresis, tinnitus, acid-base disturbances
- > 300 mg/kg: Moderate/severe toxicity: N/V, lethargy, confusion, seizures, coma

*Done Nomogram starts at 6 hr post ingestion and cannot be used if:
- Acute ingestion when salicylates have been taken within the last 24 hr
- OD was ingested over several hours
- Chronic salicylate poisonings
- Ingestion of enteric coated ASA

Tx: Adult:
- Baseline labs: CBC, electrolytes, BUN, creatinine glucose, PT, PTT, ABG, toxicology screen
- Charcoal 50 – 60 g
- NaHCO$_3$ 1 mEq/kg IV bolus until serum pH is at least 7.5

(con't)

Salicylate Toxicity (con't)

- Alkaline diuresis: 0.5 – 1.0 mEq/kg/L of NaHCO$_3$ w/ 20 – 40 mEq KCl/L in D$_5$W @ 2 – 3 times maintenance for a target urinary pH of 7 – 8
- Hemodialysis for blood levels in excess of 100 – 130 mg/dl
- Vitamin K for prolonged PT
- Frequent monitoring (q 2 hr) of ABG's, serum electrolytes and urine pH
  *Small Δ's in serum K$^+$ or arterial pH can have a dramatic effect on the degree of toxicity and salicylate clearance

Tx: Peds:
- Multiple doses of activated charcoal 1 g/kg w/ sorbitol
- D$_5$LR @ 20 ml/kg/hr × 1 – 2 hr until adequate UO
- 1 – 2 mEq/kg NaHCO$_3$ IV
- NaHCO$_3$ gtt: Mix 3 ampules of 44 mEq NaHCO$_3$ in 1 L D$_5$W w/ 20 – 40 mEq KCl/L and infuse at 1.5 – 2.0 times maintenance to obtain UO of 2 ml/kg/hr
- Vitamin K IV prn based on coagulation studies
- Administer glucose if patient has s/s of hypoglycemia even if wnl serum glucose levels

- Hemodialysis for unresponsive acidosis, hepatic failure, renal failure, pulmonary edema, persistent mental status changes or progressive clinical deterioration

- - - - - - - - - - - - - - - - - - - -

TRICYCLIC ANTIDEPRESSANT OVERDOSE

- TCA's stimulate catecholamine release and block reuptake
- Central and peripheral anticholinergic actions (delirium, mydriasis)
- Quinidine-like membrane stabilizing effect
- Direct α-blocking actions

S/S:

- Anticholinergic: confusion, delirium, anxiety, sz, coma, vasodilation, tachycardia, hyperpyrexia, mydriasis, urinary retention, $\downarrow$ GI motility, $\downarrow$ secretions
- Inhibition of α-Receptors: hypotension, reflex tachycardia, miosis
- GABA Antagonism: sz
- Na$^+$ Channel Blockade: prolongation of PR and QRS, heart blocks, $\downarrow$ myocardial contractility, hypotension, ectopy, pulmonary edema, cardiogenic shock

(con't)

TCA Overdose (con't)
- K$^+$ Channel Antagonist: QT interval prolongation
- ECG: terminal 40 msec QRS axis > 120°

Tx: Adult:
  Alkalinization:
  - ↓ free, nonprotein bound form of tricyclic molecule
  - Overrides tricyclic induced Na$^+$ channel blockade of phase 1 action potential
  - Use for patients w/ QRS > 100 ms, ventricular arrhythmias, hypotension unresponsive to 500 – 1000 ml NS bolus
    - Raise pH to 7.45 – 7.55 w/ 1 mEq/kg NaHCO$_3$ over 1 – 2 min
      *ABG for confirmation
    - NaHCO$_3$ gtt: 100 mEq NaHCO$_3$ in 0.45% NS or D$_5$W @ 2 ml/kg/hr or 150 – 200 ml/hr until QRS < 100 ms, arrhythmias cease or normotension returns
    - Maintain pH 7.45 – 7.55 w/ ABG confirmation

Magnesium:
- If QT prolonged or Torsades, give 2 g IV bolus if unstable or over 1 – 5 min if hemodynamically stable
  *Up to 5 – 10 g IV may be given

Cardiac Arrest:
- PEA
  - Hyperventilation
  - $NaHCO_3$ infusion to a pH of 7.50 – 7.55
  - NS @ > 1000 ml/hr
  - Epinephrine if alkalinization and NS infusion $\varnothing$ immediately reverse patients status

- Ventricular ectopy/ VT (if stable)
  - Alkalinization
  - Lidocaine 1.0 – 1.5 mg/kg
  - Lidocaine gtt
  - Mg^{++} 2 g over 1 – 5 min
  - Phenytoin 25 – 50 mg/min
  *$\varnothing$ use procainamide due to TCA like effects

(con't)

343

TCA Overdose – Tx Adult (con't)
- VF
    - Defib 200 J, 300 J, 360 J
    - Intubate, O_2, hyperventilate
    - Epinephrine 1.0 mg IV bolus
    - $NaHCO_3$ 1.0 mEq/kg IV bolus
    - Lidocaine 1.5 mg/kg IV bolus
    - Bretylium 500 mg IV bolus
    - Mg^{++} 2 g IV bolus
    - Repeat lidocaine 0.5 mg/kg IV bolus

Defibrillate after each medication

Tx: Peds
- ABC's
- Sz: Benzodiazepines and phenobarbital
  ∅ use phenytoin – arrhythmias
- Cardiac symptoms
    - $1 - 2$ mEq/kg $NaHCO_3$ to keep pH > 7.45

    OR
    - $NaHCO_3$ gtt: Mix 3 ampules of 44 mEq $NaHCO_3$ in 1 L D_5W w/ $20 - 40$ mEq KCl/L and infuse at $1.5 - 2.0$ times maintenance to obtain UO of 2 ml/kg/hr
- Charcoal w/ sorbitol 1 g/kg

- - - - - - - - - - - - - - - - - -

TRAUMA / BURN / ENVIRONMENTAL

BURNS

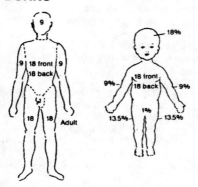

(From Guckeyson, K; Pasztor, B: *St. Vincent & Medical College LifeFlight/Mobile Life Critical Care Transport Network Pocket Emergency Guide*, 2nd ed., St. Vincent Medical Center, 1993)

Critical Burns Requiring Burn Center Management:
- 3° burns > 10% BSA
- Burns (any degree) totaling > 30% BSA
- Burns w/ respiratory injury
- Electrical burns
- Most burns involving the face, hands, feet or genitalia
- Burns associated w/ multiple trauma/fractures

(con't)

345

Burns (con't)
Baxter-Parkland Formula
4 ml × % burn × kg wt = IVF over first 24 hr

*Use LR for the first 24 hrs
*Give ½ in first 8 hr; remaining ½ in next 16 hr

Second 24 hrs
- D_5W @ 1 ml × kg wt × % burn to maintain UO at 0.5 – 1.0 ml/kg/hr
- Albumin
  - 30 – 50% burn: 0.3 ml/kg/% burn
  - 50 – 70% burn: 0.4 ml/kg/% burn
  - > 70% burn: 0.5 ml/kg/% burn

- -

DROWNING/NEAR-DROWNING
Drowning: Death due to submersion in water or within a 24 hr period

Near-Drowning: Immersion event requiring medical treatment in which the patient survives for > 24 hr, regardless of eventual outcome

*Regardless of the tonicity of the water, clinically important electrolyte abnormalities, fluid shifts and changes in Hct are unusual in near-drowning patients

*Hypovolemic shock is common and is due to hypoxic damage to the vessels which causes third spacing

Tx Goal: Improve tissue oxygen delivery as quickly as possible in order to minimize cerebral hypoxia and ischemia

Tx: Supportive care
- ABC's w/ c-spine control
- Treat hypothermia
- Endotracheal intubation and ventilation w/ PEEP
- Bronchospasm: bronchodilators
- Antibiotics for documented infection ONLY
- Manage metabolic acidosis
- BP support
- Cerebral edema
    - Hyperventilate to an $ETCO_2$ of 25 mmHg
    - Mannitol 1 – 2 g/kg IV q 3 – 4 hr
    - Furosemide 1 mg/kg IV q 4 – 6 hr

*Usually < 5 ml/kg of fluid has been aspirated
*Respiratory deterioration can be seen up to 72 hr after the near-drowning incident and is due to secondary drowning, ARDS, chemical pneumonitis, pneumonia

- -

ELECTROCUTION

Tx: Adult:
- ABC's w/ c-spine control
- O_2, monitor, IV
- Fluid replacement per burn protocol
- Myoglobinuria:
    - Maintain UO 50 – 100 ml/hr w/ LR or NS
    - Alkalinize urine: 0.5 – 1.0 mEq/kg/L of $NaHOC_3$ in D_5W
        - Maintain UO 1.0 – 1.5 ml/kg/hr OR
        - Blood pH $\geq$ 7.45
    - Mannitol 25 g initial bolus followed by 12.5 g/hr

Tx: Peds: Follow burn protocol and maintain UO 0.5 – 2.0 ml/kg/hr

- -

GLASCOW COMA SCALE (GCS) – ADULT

1. **Eye Opening**

Spontaneously	4
To Verbal Response	3
To Pain	2
No Response	1

2. **Verbal Response**

Oriented	5
Confused	4
Inappropriate Words	3
Incomprehensible Words	2
None	1

3. **Motor Response**

Obeys Commands	6
Localizes Pain	5
Withdraws from Pain	4
Abnormal Flexion	3
Abnormal Extension	2
None	1

Total GCS = Score 1 + Score 2 + Score 3

*Localize Pain: Use midline stimulus, i.e. sternal rub, orbital rim pain
*Withdraw to Pain: Use peripheral stimulus, i.e. pain nailbeds

- -

GLASCOW COMA SCALE (MGCS) – MODIFIED FOR PEDIATRICS

Score	Infant (Preverbal)	Child
Eye Opening:		
4	Opens eyes spontaneously	Opens eyes spontaneously
3	Opens eyes to speech	Opens eyes to speech
2	Opens eyes to pain	Opens eyes to pain
1	No response	No response
Verbal Response:		
5	Coos, babbles, cries appropriately	Oriented, appropriate use of words
4	Irritable cry	Confused
3	Cries only to pain	Inappropriate use of words
2	Moans to pain	Incomprehensive words
1	No response	No response
Motor Response:		
6	Spont. movements	Obeys commands
5	Withdraws to touch	Localizes pain (purposeful mvt)
4	Withdraws from pain	Withdraws from pain
3	Abnormal flexion	Abnormal flexion
2	Abnormal extension	Abnormal extension
1	No response	No response

Total GCS = Score 1 + Score 2 + Score 3

- - - - - - - - - - - - - - - - - - - -

HEAT STROKE/HYPERTHERMIA

- ABC's w/ intubation if unconscious or supplemental O_2 if not
- Remove clothing
- Immediately splash w/ fluids
- IV w/ NS or LR @ 250 ml/hr
  *Less in elderly or patients w/ CHF
- Foley
- Monitor core temperature and ECG

Temperature > 41°C (106°F)

- Ice packs to the axilla and groin
- Spray or sponge tepid (NOT cold) H_2O on the undressed patient w/ fans blowing on the patient
  *Fans must be positioned close to the patient
  *Provides the safest, quickest way to ↓ temperature
  *∅ cover w/ wet sheets – ↓ heat loss
- Cool gastric lavage if the patient is intubated
- Cool peritoneal lavage – effective and rapid @ core cooling
- Cool until core temperature is 40°C (104°F)

*Shivering is provoked at skin temperature of 28 – 33°C

- ↑ heat output up to nine-fold by ↓ heat loss through vasoconstriction
- WILL ↑ the core temperature during cooling measures

351 (con't)

Heat Stroke/Hyperthermia (con't)

Tx:

- Hypotension
    - Fluid challenge
    - Cooling
    - Dopamine as last resort

- Shivering
    - Benzodiazepines are first choice
    - Chlorpromazine 25 – 50 mg IV
      *Will lower sz threshold
    - Thiopental

- Sz
    - Diazepam 5 – 10 mg IV
    - Phenobarbital 130 – 260 mg IV
      *MR PRN

Complications: Death, cardiogenic shock,
liver failure, renal failure,
neurologic damage,
coagulopathies, electrolyte
abnormalities, rhabdomyolysis

– – – – – – – – – – – – – – – – – – – –

HYPOTHERMIA

- ABC's w/ intubation if unconscious or supplemental O_2 if not
- Remove wet garments and replace w/ blankets and insulating blankets
- Avoid rough movement
- Monitor core temperature and ECG

If pulse and breathing are present:
- **Mild hypothermia (34 – 36°C)**
    - Passive rewarming
    - Active external rewarming

- **Moderate hypothermia (30 – 34°C)**
    - Passive rewarming
    - Active external rewarming of trunk only

- **Severe hypothermia (< 30°C)**
    - Active internal warming
        - Warm IV fluids
        - Warm humidified O_2
        - Peritoneal lavage
        - *Must be KCl free
        - Warm gastric lavage
        - Extracorporeal rewarming

(con't)

Hypothermia (con't)
If pulse and breathing are absent:
- Start CPR
- Defibrillate VF/Pulseless VT 200 J, 300 J, 360 J
  *No > 3 shocks
- Intubate and ventilate w/ warm humidified O_2
- Establish IV w/ warm NS fluids

- **Core Temperature < 30°C**
  - Continue CPR
  - Withhold IV medications
  - Continue w/ active rewarming until core temperature > 35°C, return of spontaneous circulation or cessation of resuscitative measures

- **Core Temperature > 30°C**
  - Continue CPR
  - IV medications as indicated but at longer intervals
  - Repeat defibrillation for VF/Pulseless VT as core temperature ↑
  - Continue w/ active rewarming until core temperature > 35°C, return of spontaneous circulation or cessation of resuscitative measures

- - - - - - - - - - - - - - - - - - - -

HYPOVOLEMIC SHOCK

Class I
- EBL: < 750 ml (up to 15%)
- HR: < 140
- RR: 14 – 20
- BP: wnl
- PP: wnl to ↑

Class II
- EBL: 750 – 1500 ml (15 – 30%)
- HR: > 100
- RR: 20 – 30
- BP: wnl
- PP: ↓

Class III
- EBL: 1500 – 2000 ml (30 – 40%)
- HR: > 120
- RR: 30 – 40
- BP: ↓
- PP: ↓

Class IV
- EBL: > 2000 ml
- HR: > 140
- RR: > 35
- BP: ↓
- PP: ↓

EBL: estimated blood loss, PP: pulse pressure

(con't)

Hypovolemic Shock (con't)
Goals
- Primary Goal: Maintain CO
- Secondary Goal: Correct Hct w/ PRBC

Endpoints of Volume Resuscitation
- CVP > 15 mmHg
- PCWP 10 – 12 mmHg
- CI > 3 L/min/m^2
- O$_2$ Uptake (Vo$_2$) > 100 ml/min/m^2
- Lactic acid < 4 mmol/L
- Base deficit – 3 to +3 mmol/L

NOTE: Fluid replacement is 3:1 of crystalloid to colloid since only 25 – 30% of the crystalloid infused will stay in the intravascular space

*Administration of PRBC's may ↑ tissue O$_2$ deficit and ↓ blood flow due to ↑ the viscosity of the intravascular space

- - - - - - - - - - - - - - - - - - - -

356

PEDIATRIC TRAUMA SCORE (PTS)

	+2	+1	-1
Size	> 20 kg	10 – 20 kg	< 10 kg
Airway	Normal	Maintained	Unmaintained
SBP	> 90	50 – 90	< 50
CNS	Awake	Obtunded	Coma
Open Wound	None	Minor	Major
Skeletal	None	Closed	Open/Multiple

Total Points _____

*Circle one variable (+2, +1, -1) from each line and add together to obtain total points

- -

REVISED TRAUMA SCORE (RTS), ADULT

	Value	Points
A. Respiratory Rate	10 – 29	4
	> 29	3
	6 – 9	2
	1 – 5	1
	0	0
B. Systolic Blood Pressure	89	4
	76 – 89	3
	50 – 75	2
	1 – 49	1
	0	0

C. GLASGOW COMA SCALE (GCS)

1. Eye Opening

Spontaneously	4
To Verbal Response	3
To Pain	2
No Response	1

2. Verbal Response

Oriented	5
Confused	4
Inappropriate Words	3
Incomprehensible Words	2
None	1

3. Motor Response

Obeys Commands	6
Purposeful Movement (Pain)	5
Withdrawal (Pain)	4
Flexion (Pain)	3
Extension (Pain)	2
None	1

Total GCS = C
12 – 15 = 4 points
 9 – 11 = 3 points
 6 – 8 = 2 points
 4 – 5 = 1 point
   3   = 0 points

TOTAL POINTS: A + B + C = RTS

TRAUMA ALERT/
PRIORITY/CONSULT – ADULT

Trauma Alert
- Intubated
- Shock SBP < 90 documented by transport crew
- Penetrating injury to head, neck, trunk, upper thigh
- Witnessed unconsciousness OR GCS motor score < 5 (localizes pain)
- Revised Trauma Score (RTS) < 11
- Burns > 50% BSA or any trauma w/ burns or burns w/ airway compromise

(con't)

Trauma A/P/C – Adult (con't)
Trauma Priority
- Potentially unstable or deteriorating airway
- Persistent HR > 100
- History of LOC with GCS 9 – 14
- Multiple injuries
- Burns > 20%

    - Consider Trauma Priority if:
        - Ejection from auto
        - Dead passenger in same auto
        - Falls > 20 feet w/ injuries
        - Auto vs pedestrian w/ injuries
        - Motorcycle accident w/ injuries
        - Prolonged extrication
        - Hypothermia < 34.4°C
        - Child abuse

Trauma Consult
- Injury is 1° or 2° diagnosis w/
    - Stable vital signs
    - Patient is conscious
    - RTS 11 – 12
    - Admitted burns < 20%

- - - - - - - - - - - - - - - - - - - -

TRAUMA ALERT/ CONSULT/PRIORITY – PEDIATRIC

Trauma Alert
- Respiratory distress
- Shock
- Neurological injury
    - GCS < 9
    - GCS motor score < 5
    - ↓ LOC or persistent unconsciousness
    - Acute traumatic paralysis
- Traumatic injuries
    - Penetrating injury to the head, neck, trunk or upper thigh
    - Burns > 20% BSA and/or smoke inhalation
    - Vascular injuries proximal to the elbows or knees
    - Limb threatening injuries

(con't)

Trauma A/P/C – Pediatric (con't)
Trauma Priority
- No s/s shock
- Witnessed LOC or GCS 9 – 14
- ≥ 2 long bone fractures
- Blunt abdominal trauma w/ rigidity, tenderness or "seatbelt" sign
- High suspicion of a c-spine injury

    - Consider Trauma Priority if:
        - Ejection from auto
        - Dead passenger in same auto
        - Falls > 20 feet w/ injuries
        - Auto vs pedestrian w/ injuries
        - Motorcycle accident w/ injuries
        - Prolonged extrication
        - Hypothermia < 34.4°C
        - Child abuse

Trauma Consult
- Admitted burns < 20%
- Injury is a 1° or 2° diagnosis
- Isolated/single system injury w/
    - Stable vital signs
    - Conscious

- -

TRIAGE GUIDELINES FOR TRANSPORT TO A TRAUMA CENTER

Clinical Guidelines:
1. GCS ≤ 12, RTS < 11, Pediatric Trauma Score < 9 or ↓ LOC
2. SBP ≤ 90 mmHg (adults)
3. Respiratory rate < 10 or > 29 (adults)
4. Penetrating trauma to head, neck, torso
5. Flail chest
6. > 2 long bone fractures
7. Pelvic fracture(s)
8. Limb paralysis
9. Amputation proximal to the wrist or ankle

Other Factors to be Considered:
1. Ejection from vehicle
2. Death in same passenger compartment
3. Extrication time > 20 min
4. Falls > 20 feet
5. Roll over accident
6. High speed crash
7. Auto vs. pedestrian / auto vs. bicycle w/ impact @ > 5 mph

(con't)

Trauma Guidelines for Transport to a Trauma Center (con't)

8. Motorcycle accident @ > 20 mph w/ rider separated from cycle
9. Previous cardiac or respiratory dz, diabetes, cirrhosis, morbid obesity
10. Pregnancy
11. Immunosuppressed patients
12. Patients w/ known bleeding disorders

- - - - - - - - - - - - - - - - - - - -

NOTES

NOTES

NOTES

NOTES

NOTES

INDEX

C

R

BIBLIOGRAPHY

Alario, Anthony, <u>Practical Guide to the Care of the Pediatric Patient</u>, Mosby-Year Book, Inc., 1997.

American College of Surgeons, <u>Advanced Trauma Life Support</u>, 1994.

American Heart Association, <u>Advanced Cardiac Life Support</u>, 1997.

American Heart Association, <u>Inspection and Palpation of Venous and Arterial Pulses</u>, 1990.

American Heart Association, <u>Neonatal Resuscitation</u>, 1994.

American Heart Association, <u>Pediatric Advanced Life Support</u>, 1994.

Aminoff, Michael, et.al., <u>Clinical Neurology</u>, 3rd ed., Appleton et Lange, 1996.

Bakerman, Seymour, <u>ABC's of Interpretive Laboratory Data</u>, 3rd ed., Interpretive Laboratory Data, 1994.

Barken, R. & Rosen, P.; <u>Emergency Pediatrics: A Guide to Ambulatory Care</u>, Mosby, 1999.

Brose, John, et. al.; <u>The Pocket Guide to EKG Interpretation</u>, Ohio University College of Osteopathic Medicine, 1993.

Brunner, Lillian Sholtis, Suddarth, Doris Smith, et. Al., <u>Textbook of Medical-Surgical Nursing</u>, 6th ed., J.B. Lippincott Company, Philadelphis, 1988.

Campbell, John E.; <u>Basic Trauma Life Support</u>, Prentiss-Hall, 1995.

Carey, Charles et al., <u>The Washington Manual of Medical Therapeutics</u>, 29th ed., Lippincott-Raven, 1998.

Ferri, Fred F., <u>Practical Guide to the Care of the Medical Patient</u>, 4th ed., Mosby, Inc., 1998

Fix, James D.; <u>High Yield Neuroanatomy</u>, Williams & Wilkins, 1995.

Gomella, Leonard G., et. al; <u>Clinician's Pocket Reference</u>, 8th ed., Appleton & Lange, 1997.

Guckeyson, K., Pasztor, BJ., <u>Life Flight/Mobile Life Pocket Emergency Guide</u>, 2nd ed., 1993.

<u>Harrison's Principles of Internal Medicine Companion Handbook</u>, 13th ed., McGraw-Hill, Inc., St. Louis, 1995.

Lederman, Robert; <u>Internal Medicine and Critical Care Pocketbook</u>, Tarascon Publishing, Loma Linda, CA, 1997.

Lee, Genell; <u>Flight Nursing Principles and Practice</u>, Mosby Year Book, St. Louis, 1991.

Marino, Paul L., <u>The ICU Book</u>, 2nd ed., Williams & Wilkins, 1998.

Mercier, Lonnie R.; <u>Practical Orthopedics</u>, 4th ed., Mosby-Year Book Inc., 1995.

<u>Mosby's Dictionary: Medical, Nursing & Allied Health,</u> 3rd ed., C.V. Mosby Company, St. Louis, 1990.

Nelson, Waldo, et.al., <u>Textbook of Pediatrics</u>, 15th ed., W.B. Saunders Company, 1996.

<u>Nursing98 Drug Handbook</u>, Springhouse Corporation, 1998.

Nwariaku, F. & Thal, E.; <u>Parkland Trauma Handbook</u>, Mosby, 2nd ed., C.V, Mosby Company, 1999.

<u>Physicians' Desk Reference 2000</u>, Medical Economics Company, Inc., 1999.

Rogers, Mark, et. al., <u>Textbook of Pediatric Intensive Care</u>, 3rd ed., Lippincott, Williams & Wilkins, 1996.

Scott, James R. et al., <u>Danforth's handbook of Obstertics and Gynecology</u>, Lippincott-Raven, 1996.

Siberry, G. & Iannone, R.; <u>The Harriet Lane Handbook</u>, 15th ed., Mosby-Year Book, Inc., 2000.

Siedel, Henry M., et. al.; <u>Mosby's Guide to Physical Examination</u>, 3rd ed., Mosby-Year Book Inc., 1996.

<u>The Merck Manual</u>, 16th ed., Merck & Co., Inc., 1992.

Tintinalli, Judith E., et. al.; <u>Emergency Medicine: A Comprehensive Study Guide</u>, McGraw-Hill Companies, Inc., 1996.